RELATIONAL REFLEXOLOGY SUPPO' ... 'LIENTS

A PRACTITIONER GUIDE

NICHOLA GREGORY BA (HONS)

Medical Disclaimer:

The information contained in this book is not intended to serve as a replacement for professional medical advice. Any use of the information in this book is at the reader's discretion. The author and publisher specifically deny any and all liability arising directly or indirectly from the use or application of any information contained in this book. A health care professional should always be consulted regarding your specific situation.

First Printing, 2013

ISBN-13: 978-1489569523

ISBN-10: 1489569529

CONTENTS

ACKNOWLEDGMENTS

This book is dedicated to every woman who has trusted me with her innermost fears and struggles *and* allowed me to share in much deserved moments of achievement and joy. Special thanks in particular to each of the women represented in both the case study chapter and in the women's words sections. Without your generous contributions this book would not exist. I am indebted to you all.

Thanks also to my friends and colleagues who have continued to support and encourage me throughout this project. I am grateful for the editing and the willing ears. Particular thanks must go to Christine McCluskey and Jackie Pounder for their creative teaching methods and non-judgmental attitude, without which I would have been unable to construct this text. Thanks also go to Juliet Wilson for helping me to define and clarify, and to Rosie March-Smith for her wonderfully generous time and encouragement.

To my beautiful son Cameron, thank you for your never-ending patience through many hours of writing and for being my eternal, smiling sunshine.

FOREWORD

Mention the word reflexology to anyone in the medical profession and it will evoke much the same dismissive raised eyebrow as if you had said ectoplasm or Atlantis. The fact that foot massage as a subtle form of healing was practiced thousands of years ago in Ancient Egypt will probably be as much lost on them as the equally significant fact of the use of acupuncture techniques in China, also millennia ago. Yet both are still around (and in the Western world), even though their once revered status has long since diminished.

Whom should we blame for this current bad image? Unfortunately, some of the present day scepticism is due to prejudice and ignorance: this latter sometimes thanks to those people who decide one fine morning to find employment in the 'alternative healing' world. They learn their 'skills' in the briefest of weekend trainings, hurry to advertise their services the following week and are likely then to become accidentally responsible for serious unprofessional conduct. Boundary blurring, forming casual sexual relationships with clients, offering directive advice (with dangerous consequences), these misdemeanours seem of little concern to such sloppy people. We've all heard about their behaviour and are powerless to stop it - unless, that is, they have an accrediting body who can insist they cease practice.

Fortunately, there are highly trained, professionally rigourous practitioners *also* out there. And it is to encourage more of them that this book, along with its accompanying training scheme, is now introduced. The book's gifted author Nichola Gregory is not only herself a prime example of such rigorous training, but she has had the courage to declare herself in print to insist on the raising of standards professionally in her chosen field.

As a relational reflexologist working in private practice she is in an ideal position to persuade students to take the long, hard road to real qualification. Their certificate of accreditation will mean a true measure of expertise, ensuring that graduates take with them into their new practice a level of integrity and education bearing no comparison with those 'weekend' trainees still plying their trade out there. Nichola's passionate belief in improving both the standards of practice in reflexology *per se*, but also in training practitioners specifically who work with clients with sub-fertility issues, shine through this book. Recognising the vulnerability of such women, the need for extreme care in honouring ethical responsibility to them, is clearly a primary concern of hers. She is rightly angry about the irresponsibility of the 'weekend qualifiers', where their self-importance and unrealistic promises to their clients can cause such emotional damage. Movingly describing the isolation women feel when they have difficulty in conceiving a longed-for child, their bewilderment and distress, Nichola writes with great compassion and she uses their reported words in one chapter to great effect. She writes too of clinical, psychological and medical matters in a manner both clear and helpful.

This is not only a thoughtful book, it is a timely one. Her fascinating research into the rise and fall of the ancient healing arts, where Christianity dealt them a near-terminal blow in the Middle Ages, compounded by scientists in later centuries, who nearly (but not quite) wiped esoteric knowledge off the board, is traced compellingly.

That titanic clash between science and the ancient healing arts is, however, at long last beginning a new phase. Tentative it may be, but far more accepting of others' views, now that consciousness is coming more to the fore again. We have complementary therapy as part of our twenty first century lexicon, where qualified practitioners in all alternative disciplines are sometimes welcome to work in tandem with modern medicine. This is a good enough compromise to be going on with, each side actually acknowledging the value of the other. More doctors than ever appear to be accepting alternative healing methods (Chinese medical herbs; acupuncture; osteopathy; homeopathy; reflexology and so on), either because they are finally enlightened or overworked, or a bit of both. All this despite the anti-lobby, unhelpful whatever their rationale, be it political, fiscal or expedient. I believe there is hope for the future, when appropriate national registration and accreditation in all fields of complementary therapy will give more confidence to orthodox medical practitioners and thence the general public.

But that hope for a more holistic approach to healing cannot become a reality unless and until complementary therapies are given the status they deserve. How do practitioners achieve such status? By embarking on a proper education for them and preparing to meet demanding criteria in their chosen healing discipline.

Here I would flag up my personal crusade: to encourage students in all complementary therapies to learn basic listening skills, sign on for a foundation course (at the very least) in counselling from an accredited training body, and to follow Nichola's own lead in taking her earlier studies to the next level.

May her book inspire students to do just that, ultimately to contribute *their* excellent professionalism to the entire field of complementary therapy.

Rosie March-Smith

INTRODUCTION

My working life as a complementary therapist began in 2005 when I initially trained in reflexology and auricular acupuncture. Fairly soon into practice I became aware that despite being initially guided towards encouraging silence in the consulting room, my reflexology clients didn't always wish to adhere to such a *rule*. It wasn't long before I found myself enrolling on an entry level counselling course, eventually graduating as a professional counsellor in 2010. Since 2006 I have worked with over 150 sub-fertility clients.

My greatest hope for this book is that it will go some way towards raising current professional standards in reflexology, and help to protect vulnerable client groups from uninformed practice. The book is not constructed to furnish the reader with a new routine or technique. I have deliberately chosen not to reference any specific reflexology points or to concentrate on the physical application of reflexology. Rather the intention with the book is to guide those more experienced practitioners as they develop a sound professional rationale for their reflexology practice and a deeper appreciation of what might be happening within the confines of their reflexology consulting rooms. Practitioners wishing to engage with vulnerable client groups are ethically required to be already familiar and competent in the application of their particular physical form of reflexology practice.

The recent adoption of reflexology by the beauty and spa industry has unfortunately resulted in rapidly declining standards of education and an over simplified theoretical comprehension of the potential impact of the modality. When I completed my own reflexology training in 2005 the course entailed over 100 hours of direct teaching across a 12 month period, 60 full case study presentations *(the file was bigger than my degree dissertation)* and the requirement to complete a separate pre-requisite diploma in A&P.

Today, a 'practitioner' can walk away with a certificate stating qualification in reflexology in as little as two days! In our modern world of standardisation and litigation, now more than ever before, the responsibility of protecting reflexology and its reputation falls directly on the shoulder of every professional reflexology practitioner. It is vital professional practitioners are able to validate and rationalise their stance of practice, particularly in the UK, where recent changes to advertising regulations mean practitioners are finding their modality claims to be increasingly in the spotlight.

Encouragingly for the professional relational reflexologist there already exists a large and robust body of academic and clinical information supporting the ethical and informed application of complementary modalities such as reflexology. This book presents a rationale for professional practice built upon that information.

As well as containing clinical information relating to sub-fertility, IVF protocols and scientific research and hypothesis linked to the principles of psychoneuroimmunology, the book also contains an extensive chapter exploring the concept of the therapeutic relationship in reflexology, and examines how such a relationship might be impacting on reflexology clients.

To provide context I have included a chapter of qualitative type reflective case studies and two sections of women's words. The case studies are taken from practice, anonomised, and have been presented in as verbatim a manner as possible in an attempt to minimise bias. Towards the end of the book I have included a brief chapter introducing the basic principle of TCM (Traditional Chinese Medicine) for the reader's information.

Throughout the book I have tried to impress upon the reader the huge ethical responsibility existing for those practitioners who wish to engage with sub-fertility clients, or indeed any vulnerable client group. There are probably few reflexologists who have not at some time taken a phone call or received an email from a client enquiring about reflexology to support sub-fertility. Women's magazines, internet support forums and word of mouth continue to advertise and champion the potential benefits of reflexology, but how many practitioners are able to explain or rationalise their reflexology interventions?

It is quite simply not acceptable to offer hope without reason to emotionally vulnerable client groups, and the sub-fertility group is perhaps amongst the most vulnerable. These often distressed, anxious women are deserving of not only the gentlest of care and touch from their reflexology practitioners, but also of the highest professional standards and levels of informed practitioner knowledge.

Sub-fertility clients metaphorically walk into the reflexology consulting room and place their hopes and dreams in the practitioner's hands. The role of the professional supportive relational reflexologist is not only to touch and care, but also to gently refuse that offered *power* with the relationship and to strive instead to encourage client autonomy and self directed change.

Professional reflexology practitioners are not magicians; we certainly do NOT get women pregnant! This is a vitally important stance for practitioners to adopt, not only in order to promote client autonomy and self directed change, but also to ensure increased development of professional relationships with the general medical and psychological community.

If by the end of this book the reader feels additional training might be required to ensure excellence of practice, then that can only be good news for this vulnerable group of women already regularly sourcing reflexology support.

Terminology

Aware of the prevalence of female practitioners I have tried to avoid gender bias where possible. Throughout the book I use the term practitioner (and sometimes therapist) to represent the reflexologist and client to represent the receiver.

CHAPTER ONE

ANCIENT PERSPECTIVES AND MODERN MEDICINE

The concept of ancient health and medicine can sometimes appear mysterious and difficult to comprehend to modern day human beings, particularly if attempts are made to measure the Ancient's knowledge by today's intellectual, scientific models and standards. The formation and growth of modern medicine can be traced back across thousands of years. Its development encouraged by more settled human societies, religion, philosophy, education, trade and of course the ever enquiring human mind. Latterly with so many astonishing advances occurring within science and modern medicine it is perhaps easy to imagine human beings could only have gained with regards to their health. Whilst scientific achievements are undoubtedly of tremendous value to the entire human race, it could be argued along its developmental journey both science and modern medicine became a little blinded to fully appreciating the complex human condition and the innate and subtle interactions of mind and body.

Pre-History

Pre-literate man left us no written record of his knowledge of the body, health or medicines, although anthropologists have been able to make some associations with modern-day cultures such as the Australian Aborigines, who until the late eighteenth century remained entirely isolated from the outside world yet were discovered to be healthy (Graham, 1999). It is believed many pre-historic tribes believed in *animism*. A concept stating that individual lives and the functions of the human body were influenced by, and at the mercy of, unpredictable spirits. Belief systems such as these placed the Shaman, or witch doctor, at the centre of tribal nomadic life. The Shaman was viewed as a master of divination, healing, foresight, and interpretation. The Shaman could communicate with the spirit world. He possessed mastery over fire and rain, and could *journey* in varying altered states of consciousness for the purpose of diagnosis, prophecy or insight. Whereas in the modern sense illness and disease might be viewed as external agents affecting the body, to these ancient pre-historic and shamanic cultures illness was viewed as a spiritual matter essentially. One principally thought to stem from a loss of individual personal power and where *dis-ease* was considered as originating and gaining meaning from the spiritual.

Ancient Egypt

The emergence of the great human civilisations and the growing exploration of the wider world meant a more structured concept of healing began to emerge. The ancient Egyptians were perhaps the first to embrace and formalise the concept of medicine and healing. The Egyptian understanding of health might be likened to a middle point between pre-historic nomadic attitudes and those of the later great Greek civilisations.

Increased stability stemming from more settled farming economies encouraged the development of formalised governments, laws and social norms, as well as sparking the emergence of structured religious practices and the invention of writing and calculation. The significant development of writing was important as rather than relying on verbal tradition alone for passing on knowledge ideas could be now be recorded and developed for further study and education.

Medicine however was still deeply rooted in the magical and the divine and the healer priests of the time were highly regarded as the holders and keepers of ancient sacred wisdom. The Egyptians viewed their very existence as being intrinsically connected to the workings of the universe, and often directly to the working of their Gods. To the ancient Egyptians the universe existed in perfect energetic harmony with man considered a perfect microcosm and representation of that harmony.

As well as colour and rhythm existing as important healing tools, higher status priests were also said to be able to tap into and direct natural universal energies and they were particularly interested in energies emanating from the sun (or Ra). Healer priests sought to direct the energy emanating from the sun into their patient, and so practiced the passing of hands over the body in an attempt to invoke changes in the subtle etheric energy (or spiritual body). The priests believed healing energy could be absorbed into the more vital, physical elements of the individual, thus inducing a state of both spiritual and physical healing. The temple priests also made use of herbs and spices brought back by traders from all over the known world, and the practice of mummification encouraged a deeper understanding of the body and its internal organs.

The Egyptian concept of *channel theory* emerged after temple priests observed damage occurring in farmer's fields when the irrigation channels became blocked. The principle was also utilised as a source of understanding disease within the human body. The development of this more formalised theory of human health began to signify Egyptian Gods were no longer being perceived as entirely responsible for human illness, and the healer priests of the time began to strive towards finding more practical, physical interventions to restore the health of mind, body (and spirit). In ancient Egypt the first depictions of ***foot massage*** as a therapeutic endeavour were discovered in a painting at the tomb of Ankhmahor at Saqqara, dated circa 2300 BC, and appear to depict temple priests unblocking energetic body channels.

Ancient Greece

The ancient Greek civilisations began to emerge just as the Egyptian age began to fade. Above all it might be said the Greeks liked to think. The Greeks placed importance on the concept of rational and logical thinking, striving always to understand *why* things happen. During the time of the ancient Greeks the art of philosophy prospered. The concepts of harmony, right balance and measure were of central importance to Greek philosophers and their main aim until the sixth century BC was understanding physis; *an attempt to perceive the essential and true nature of all things.*

According to Greek myth, Asclepius, son of the god Apollo and the nymph Coronis, was born from the dead body of his mother. Asclepius was raised by Chiron, a centaur, who was considered a master of medical practice and herbal medicine. Soon Asclepius surpassed his master's knowledge and became known as the Greek God of medicine. Over 200 temples to Asclepius's were constructed representing the first known hospitals. Patients were allowed to rest and to sleep in the temples, where it was believed through dreams they might perceive the presence of the God Asclepius, who would provide therapeutic guidance and the ability to recover.

Greek philosophers during this time considered man's health to lie centrally within the remit of their thinking with the well known philosopher Plato expressing his belief that *"the cure of the part should not be attempted without treatment of the whole"*. The ancient Greeks considered the soul (or psyche) to be a moving dynamic force which could be influenced not only to induce dis-ease, but also to restore harmony. Human problems and the physical manifestations of illness were viewed as essentially spiritual in nature; literally as '*psychopathology*' (Graham, 1999).

The ancient Greeks were keen observers of feelings and moods and emotional purging and laughter were viewed as highly therapeutic. Mythology and Greek theatre were also considered useful and necessary and used to explain the meaning of otherwise difficult concepts and to invoke and induce intense emotional responses. In essence the Greeks of the time believed the key to maintaining good health lay in achieving a balance between the spiritual and the physical elements of life. To the Greeks of this period however the Gods were still deemed to be very influential, and the Greek temple priests continued to practice a great deal of the ancient knowledge inherited from the Egyptians in their own particular form of medicine.

Mathematics

During the sixth century BC the influence of Pythagorean philosophy marked the beginning of mathematics and coding, and represents the birth of modern science and linear thinking. Pythagorean theory influenced western thinking tremendously because mathematics sits at the core of the concepts of exact and measurable truths. Within the field of medicine the first indication of the practice of human dissection occurred during the fifth century BC and represents the emergence of the scientific concepts of exploration, analysis, measurement and standardisation in health and medicine. During the 5th century BC, Hippocrates, commonly regarded as the father of modern medicine, introduced his medical *'theory of four humors and temperaments'*.

According to Hippocrates physical disorders could be viewed as conditions of disharmony existing in the *humors* of the body. Hippocrates believed the individual could be affected by many factors including thoughts and emotions; their behaviours; climate; excessive or too little physical activity; water quality and even a lack of sunlight. Hippocrates believed healing the individual involved attempting to restore equilibrium in both the psychology and external environment of the individual. He stated treatment should only occur after consideration of *attitude, environmental influences and natural remedies*, and he placed worth on the body's ability to self heal given favourable conditions. The role of physician according to Hippocrates was therefore one of serving natural law.

During the mid 5th century BC the Greek philosopher Parmenides proposed physical matter was an indestructible substance made up of tiny dead particles he coined atoms. The movement of these atoms was assumed by the ancient Greeks to originate from the spiritual, although the matter itself was viewed as somehow different and separate. Philosophers of this time now began to turn their attention away from the subject of considering physical matter and how it might be connected to human life, and began instead to lean towards more existential, spiritual and ethical considerations. Scientific thinking would now take responsibility for dissecting and measuring the nature of universal physical matter.

Christianity and the middle-ages

The emergence of Christianity and its subsequent spread across Western Europe delivered an enormous blow to man's innate, ancient connection with his own personal energetic power and intuition. Man was guided towards a belief in one omnipotent God, and the church took authority on his behalf over man. Scientists across the middle-ages, under the watchful eye of the Christian Church, continued to attempt to explain the existence of God and the nature of universe using a standardised framework drawn from the concepts of Greek scientific reasoning.

During this time a real and definite attempt was made by the Church to destroy any movement, group or individual still ingrained with any belief system associated with ancient, esoteric knowledge. The healers of the day were those infused with the secrets of oral medicinal folk traditions, commonly referred to as *witches* during the middle-ages. Evidence stemming from witch trials dating to the time suggests indeed a great deal of the knowledge possessed by these mostly women healers might be viewed as essentially shamanic in origin.

Scientific milestones

It was Copernicus (1473-1543) who first proposed the notion that the planets circled the sun, and in doing so challenged Church teachings stating the earth lay at the centre of the universe. The laws of planetary motion discovered by Kepler (1571-1630) further challenged the deeply established religious view and the final proof was eventually delivered by Galileo (1564-1642) who demonstrated that the earth did indeed revolve around the sun. Collectively this marked a time of huge collision and separation between science and religion. Man and his connection with his inner self was soon dealt a further blow of separation by Descartes (1596-1650) who suggested that mind and matter were in fact two entirely different things.

Isaac Newton (1643-1727) believed the universe to be a three-dimensional space. An immovable, constant, unchangeable place existing entirely independently of the material objects it contains. According to Newton changes in the physical world existed in a separate dimension of time, which absolute in nature, flowed in a linear sequence. Newton proposed small particles existed in this place and believed gravity to be the force which explained the movement of the particles. Newton also expressed his own personal belief that theses forces and particles were created and set in motion by God at the beginning of time.

Science now began to consider the universe and the very essence of nature itself as following an unquestionable mechanistic model, with every component of life considered explainable by a cosmic set of fixed rules governed by absolute mathematical laws and equations. Within the realm of health and medicine this period in history sparked the emergence of what we refer to today as modern medicine. In 1543, Andreas Vesalius published an important human anatomy book. In 1628, William Harvey published his research on the circulation of blood in the body, and finally the microscope; an enormously important technological advancement in medicine was invented in 1670 by Anton van Leeuwenhoek.

The separation of body and mind

By the nineteenth century science had become so entrenched in a mechanistic clockwork view of the universe that the concept of God had almost become obsolete. The advent of modern physics and the growing insistence within the scientific world that all things should be universally agreed upon as objective, physical and factual, left the field of psychology with a quite a dilemma. Traditionally known for embracing the concepts of consciousness, senses and feelings, elements which ultimately could never be measured objectively, yet still anxious to be recognised and listed as a scientific endeavor, the field of psychology turned away from the study of human emotion and psyche and instead began to concentrate on the objective study of human behavior (Graham, 1999).

Science and medicine now began to view the physical elements of the individual as existing entirely separately from the mind and psyche. The diagnosis and treatment of dis-ease and illness within Western medicine has been considered in this somewhat fragmented context since.

Modern thinking

It was the publishing of Albert Einstein's Special Theory of Relativity in 1905, closely followed by Rutherford's historic splitting of the atom in 1909, that finally pulled apart the by now established mechanical, clockwork Newtonian view of the world. According to Einstein time and space were ultimately connected and four dimensional in essence. Whereas previously time was considered as fixed and linear, Einstein's theory stated time was dynamic, able to stretch and move and absolutely and intrinsically linked to space and indeed the matter contained within.

Summary

Over time individuals have become increasingly disconnected from their own personal experience and almost entirely passive regarding their health-care. Conversely science, medicine, doctors and other healthcare workers have been encouraged to adopt a professional stance of detached authority and assumed superior knowledge.

The complex physiological and emotional relationships present within the human body were unfortunately initially judged by early science as deserving no relevant place in fact or the absolute. Instead they were dismissed almost entirely in favour of a mathematical understanding of man. Science and the medical profession have become modern day Gods and human individuals are now more detached from their own existence and personal responsibility than they have been in perhaps many thousands of years.

"The more specialized doctors become, the more they know about a body part or organ and the less they tend to understand the human being in whom that part or organ resides." (Mate, 2003).

As we will explore in more detail in chapter three, the very existence of human HPA axis (hypothalamus-pituitary-adrenal axis) means the experiences and perceptions of the individual can and do affect the physical body in a very real and direct manner. This concept unfortunately currently seems to hold little relevance within much of western allopathic medicine and is becoming alarmingly diluted in the practice of an increasingly sanitised form of holistic medicine. In the field of relational reflexology for sub-fertility a woman's perceptions and emotions, in addition to her body's reaction to them, provide the core rationale for practice.

The separation of mind and body, and indeed man from his wider experiencing, unfortunately dictates man can never truly be perceived, measured or treated as a whole. As practitioners of reflexology, or indeed any holistic modality, it seems crucial that as we move into the future we are able to retain a blend of practice which retains a truly holistic, multi-dimensional essence. Twentieth century physics suggests a basic oneness exists within our universe. These up to date scientific principles suggest we inhabit a far more complex and interactive universe than could ever have been imagined. Perhaps in the future we might come to increasingly accept this concept also applies in the consideration of human health. As Helen Graham *(1999)* correctly points out:

> *"A fundamental problem facing contemporary medicine is that of reconciling ordinary descriptions of bodies, health and disease with the idea that the universe and everything in it is an inseparable entity."*

Encouragingly the scientific field of psychoneuroimmunocrinology (PNI), a relatively young branch of research established during the early 1980s, potentially offers both allopathic and holistic researchers alike a scientific framework from which to better understand the delicate interactions between the mind, brain and endocrine and immune systems of the body. The principles of PNI and how they might be considered within the reflexology package are discussed in more depth in chapter three.

Adopting a professional stance of appreciating the *oneness* existing in our clients, through embracing both their physical and emotional being, allows the relational reflexology practitioner to engage in a more rounded and authentic holistic manner. How though might this more authentic holistic attitude be carried out in real practice? Carried out within our scientific world so focused on the measurable and absolute? The key to achieving this delicate balance lies ultimately with the individual practitioner.

Holistic: Adj.

- *Emphasising the whole and the interdependence of its parts.*
- *(Medicine) of or relating to the medical consideration of the complete person, physically and psychologically, in the treatment of a dis-ease.*

CHAPTER TWO

THE ANCIENT HEALER AND THE MODERN DAY COMPLEMENTARY THERAPIST

"As mankind evolved a place for the healer priest was heralded, a spiritual companion to accompany the traveller as he or she sought the mind-body-soul connection." (March-Smith, 2005)

The role of the healer throughout history clearly held central importance within many ancient cultures. It is perhaps interesting to reflect on how the remit of the ancient healer is not so very unlike the expectation placed upon many modern day holistic and complementary practitioners. Complementary modalities have for a long time attracted those clients often warmly referred to as medical rejects. Encouragingly more recently increasing numbers of clients seem to be sourcing complementary therapies with more preventative intentions in mind. In some cases clients may have chosen to turn away from proposed conventional medicine, for others a magazine article, internet research or perhaps a friend's referral may have sparked an interest. Often however, regardless of the initial signposting, the remit of expectation placed upon reflexology practitioners can be enormous and the boundaries of professional practice unclear.

Professional boundaries

As holistic and complementary practitioners we are recognised publicly for placing value on the interaction between mind, body (and spirit). Our initial professional training rightly guides us to be mindful of working only within our professional competencies, with reflexology principally defined as a touch and pressure therapy. Some attention may be given during the practitioner's primary training to considering the power of touch as a stand-alone therapeutic intervention, and in rare cases perhaps the nature of therapeutic relationship, but generally this is not common place.

Practitioners are taught instead how to set structured professional boundaries within their complementary therapy practice. As fledgling therapists we are often guided towards encouraging silence in the complementary treatment room and not engaging in conversation with clients. We are similarly guided towards refraining from giving any advice on diet or nutrition and instead we are recommended to follow set professional referral pathways. Through working in this structured manner initially we are of course aiming to ensure our clients remain safe and that as practitioners we work only within the realm of our professional competencies. These professional boundaries however, the foundations on which we practice, are not entirely constructed to account for the *perceived expectation* of clients. What role public might feel a practitioner holds? In the case of the sub-fertility client for example, if professional recommended referral pathways are to be strictly followed, then officially, women should be encouraged to engage not only with their supportive reflexologist, but also with a professional counsellor and a possibly even a dietician. This might be perhaps considered as rather a naive attitude emanating from a professional industry becoming increasingly ingrained within a clinical, medical model of health, and an unfortunate attitude which carries with it the assumption that clients possess both the time and financial means to engage on such a multi-therapist level.

Unfortunately neither do these initial professional boundaries, particularly when intertwined with a deep implicit fear of causing harm (and depending on the training body a potential endless list of contra-indications to delivering reflexology), actively encourage therapists to grow professionally and develop their understanding of their own therapeutic modality, theoretically and experientially.

Developing reflexology professionally

Whilst there are a few practitioners, often practicing within allied health professions and clinical settings, who may find they are asked to engage in well structured clinical type research, producing measurable data, the vast majority of reflexology practitioners are simply dealing on a day to day basis with the clients who are approaching them in private practice. Of course it is essential the profession continues to strive towards producing good quality measurable and quantifiable data relating to the specific mechanism of reflexology. However, in order to better protect and move our profession forward, it might be wise to begin actively educating and encouraging those more experienced professional practitioners working in the private sector to engage in well structured existential research studies. The results gathered could potentially yield an interesting and entirely relevant body of work. In turn this work might provide more sound justification for engaging in more detailed quantifiable or mixed methodology type research.

Scientific measurable proof is often rightly sought in areas when vulnerable people are involved. Certainly the very nature of this client group and the challenges they face both physically and emotionally would define them as vulnerable. In the field of reflexology for sub-fertility and supportive ART however, justified by facilitating precautions for safe practice, practitioners are encouraged not to undertake work with this particular client group. In reality unfortunately, for both practitioners and the general public, this has produced a professional double-edged sword.

Approached by women asking for support, yet left to work undirected and unsupported professionally because of scant clinical work available to take guidance from, in addition to the fact some key writers still openly oppose the application of reflexology during fertility treatment, practitioners are left to go it alone, and the public are left vulnerable and open to potentially poor practice. The lack of good quality CPD education, stemming from sound ethical practice is potentially harmful to the profession and the client group at risk because of poorly trained, possibly ill prepared practitioners. The professional bodies currently attempting to better regulate reflexology must acknowledge more openly the public are regularly sourcing reflexology to support their sub-fertility issues, and address the matter more pro-actively. To deny this situation exists and to continue to hide behind a lack of acceptable clinical, quantitative type research is professionally unethical and entirely unhelpful for both practitioners and the general public.

Often justification for this no-touch stance leans towards not yet understanding (scientifically) if the effects of stimulating the feet through reflexology might potentially induce in the body negative effects regarding early pregnancy and/or the effectiveness of fertility and IVF drugs.

Evidence stemming from the writers practice has demonstrated that the inclusion of supportive relational reflexology can be beneficial during an IVF protocol, with many clients reporting a reduction in commonly noted symptoms as well as demonstrating impressive IVF success rates amongst the group.

Evidence also overwhelmingly demonstrates that the application of reflexology across conception and throughout the first trimester of pregnancy will do no harm to a well structured pregnancy (see clinical observations chapter). However, as Denise Tiran offers:

> *"Loss of pregnancy occurs in 25% of pregnancies as a result of physiological or psychological factors; there is no research evidence available to confirm or deny that reflexology could cause abortion. Sadly, women who suffer miscarriage often strive to find a reason for it." (Tiran & Mackereth, 2011).*

The real fear involved in working with sub-fertility clients centres around the concept that some women who have experienced miscarriage might feel compelled to look for a reason for their loss, and may try to *blame* reflexology. It seems essential therefore the profession strives towards encouraging higher standards of professional knowledge in practitioners. This ensures such vulnerable women are cared for within ethically sound and safe reflexology environments, by professional practitioners who feel confident in understanding the real and perceived boundaries existing within the modality. Confidence in practice, underpinned by sound appropriate information reduces the chances of uneducated miscommunication occurring, as well as minimising the potential of unrealistic and unfounded expectations and fears developing in both practitioners and the wider public.

Despite these obvious professional challenges practitioners seem to be engaging in this sensitive field without any structured CPD or additional specialised training quite simply because women are asking to be supported. Perhaps this encouragingly demonstrates that that many practitioners are holding to a well documented holistic principle when they choose to *touch* their sub-fertility and ART clients; that which is pertaining to the principle of homeostasis. Perhaps too, practitioners are demonstrating that they are already utilising their own *inner supervisors* and *ethical decision making processes.*

Homeostasis: Noun

- *The tendency of a system especially the physiological system of higher animals, to maintain internal stability owing to the co-ordinated responses of its parts to any situation or stimulus that would tend to disturb its normal condition or function.*

- *Psychology. A state of psychological equilibrium obtained when tension or a drive has been reduced or eliminated.*

Ethics

The majority of women dealing with sub-fertility issues and engaging in supportive reflexology treatments are doing so within private therapy settings. Working therapeutically with clients dealing with the enormous pressures associated with sub-fertility is of course laden with huge responsibility for the complementary practitioner. For some therapists the real and assumed responsibility of being involved in something so enormous and potentially life changing means the concept of working with a woman undergoing IVF is still unimaginable to them. Certainly it might be fair to say the lack of good research and appropriate practitioner training in the field has perhaps lead to many practitioners adopting fears of potentially causing harm to the sub-fertility client or adhering to a belief that by facilitating treatment during IVF the intervention might interfere adversely with the functioning of fertility drugs.

This lack of research, and indeed the opinions currently held by some key writers within the field of reflexology pertaining to a no touch policy during ovulation or whilst a client is undertaking fertility drugs, is of course born from a desire to work ethically and professionally; above all to do no harm. The fear of somehow causing harm or of interfering with a medical intervention such as IVF is a valid one, and of course it is entirely correct to enquire as to the safety or wisdom of offering sessions. Ultimately however, the ethical decision to do so lies with the individual practitioner.

It could be argued that reflexology has become increasingly detached from its true origin as a pressure therapy traditionally utilised within a much wider healing context. An insistence within the conventional allopathic world to attempt to quantify the human experience potentially leads us as holistic therapists further away from the very nature of that we strive to practice; that being *reflexology as a therapeutic pressure therapy and interaction between two human beings both focused on the experiencing of the receiver.* This experience and any benefits resulting from it can be very difficult if not impossible to quantify according to a classical scientific paradigm. Reflexology some believe is by its very nature a holistic healing form incorporating many dimensions of experience and certainly not a medical type treatment. Perhaps then reflexology fits much more comfortably into the realm of mixed methodology or qualitatively researched enquiry?

Understanding research methodologies

Quantitative research is involved with gathering data which is absolute, such as numerical data, so it can be counted and modelled statistically. Tests are designed to remove as much bias as possible. Tests are often randomised and the information collated would be expected to remain consistent should the test be carried out repeatedly or elsewhere. This type of research is closely aligned with what is viewed as the classical scientific paradigm and might be associated with double blind trials and the use of sham reflexology points.

Qualitative research on the other hand is a much more subjective form of research enquiry. Often the data collected from a qualitative study will yield little concrete data in the form of numbers, but instead might focus on experience, stories, feelings and emotions. The researcher accepts bias as a natural part of the enquiry and that it forms a more complete picture. Studies are often presented in case study form as this allows for a richer more detailed account of the subject. The case study chapter later in this book has been constructed in a qualitative manner, primarily using the women's own words to demonstrate their personal and unique experiences of relational reflexology.

Certainly within the field of social sciences there exists enormous debate regarding the validity of qualitative studies. Some researchers feel more rigorous quantitative studies should be adopted so that results might be more generalised and gain the respect of the more scientifically minded community. Equally there are those who believe wholeheartedly that the human experience quite simply cannot be quantified.

An ideal synthesis for the future of reflexology then will perhaps be an appreciation of what *both* methodologies can bring to the development of the profession as a whole.

> *"Not all essential information can be confirmed in the laboratory or by statistical analysis. Not all aspects of illness can be reduced to facts verified by double-blind studies and by the strictest scientific techniques." (Mate, 2003).*

Leaning heavily towards understanding the exact mechanics of reflexology from a scientific, numerical, quantitative stand-point might be akin to trying to understand the taste and texture of a chocolate cake through describing its molecular structure. Whilst it might be useful to know how it's constructed, it is perhaps the taste that ultimately matters!

Fear, litigation and moving forward

During the middle ages the assumed authority of the church made a very definite attempt to destroy any movement or individual choosing to remain attached to ancient knowledge. In modern times the assumed authority has become quantifiable medicine and the fear used to gain control is litigation. Our modern world is indeed a complex and challenging one, a world in which corporate business and medicine have become perhaps uneasily intertwined and interrelated.

Medicine overwhelmingly exists as branch of science still constructed upon outdated Newtonian type viewpoints of fixed and absolute mathematical truths. Whilst quantifiable scientific enquiries undoubtedly permit us to define, focus and clarify, this form of research study should not perhaps be permitted to become the singular source of unquestionable valid empirical investigation. Science is after all an essentially fluid and ever changing exploration and one where all beginnings stem from educated empirical hypothesis. According to the general medical community however, at present, it would seem only quantitative type medical research can be acknowledged as a defining measuring tool?

To meet for example new UK ASA (advertising standards authority) required criteria, research studies must be deemed large enough to be considered valid, randomised and able to be counted and modelled statistically. Recently rulings by made the ASA mean due to a lack of 'substantive evidence' advertisers may no longer claim reflexology can 'treat, cure or diagnose' a range of medical conditions. In a document entitled 'Guidance on Health Therapies and Evidence' the ASA states:

"Our position on the acceptability and appropriateness of evidence is in line with the weight of scientific and academic opinion. We encourage professional organisations in the health therapies sector to engage with the wider scientific and academic community to develop new and rigorous methodologies that take account of the holistic nature of their therapies. Nevertheless, any new trial methodology should still have a robust basis and outcomes to ensure that the consumer can make informed decisions based on the claims made in marketing communications, which will be assessed on the basis of available scientific knowledge. We aim to ensure that our approach towards evidence and methodology is consistent across all sectors, including those outside the health sector" and that *"Advertisers must submit documentary evidence to the ASA to support any claims they make."*

Within the fields of social sciences there encouragingly already exists a very large respected and *robust* body of valid ***qualitative type*** research, principally examining the complex nature of *human experience*. Practitioners of complementary modalities such as reflexology are advised to similarly begin to define their rationale for practice, and indeed any research investigations they might collate, as primarily *qualitative* in nature. Practitioners who adopt such a theoretical stance allow for the incorporation of individual *client phenomenology* to factor in any gathered results. Practitioners adopting this attitude are also better positioned to make use of existing, valid, well documented academic and medical theoretical information and principles.

Recently formed skeptic organisations have publicly stated their intention to make use of updated ASA regulations to promote their online and real life campaign to prevent 'misleading' claims being made by complementary and holistic practitioners. Groups such as these are already bringing complaints against practitioners to the ASA and internet campaigns are underway to recruit volunteers, and it would seem sadly to attempt to generally discredit complementary medicine? Many in the complementary therapy world may be feeling a modern day 'witch hunt' is underway, however this really doesn't need to be the case.

Improving standards

In reality the guidelines recently imposed by the ASA should ultimately improve standards within our profession. Over the last decade reflexology training standards have hit an all time low. Unethical, profit driven educators offer practitioner level training to be completed in as little as two days. Our industry has been infiltrated and adopted by the beauty and spa world and as a result professional standards have dropped dramatically. As an industry we practitioners are wholly responsible for the future reputation of reflexology. We simply cannot continue in this modern world of standardisation, litigation and fear to accept such poor standards of training or to hide as an complementary industry behind what might come to pass or could be known in the future.

The growing field of psychoneuroimmunology demonstrates medicine is encouragingly finally beginning to embrace the complex and unique oneness of the human individual. However, until such a time as the modality of reflexology can be explained in more quantifiable detail practitioners must strive to ground their professional practice in educated hypothesis, ethical rationale and known fact. Reflexology training courses must therefore be more stringently constructed to prepare the professional practitioner for how to adequately meet the complex and comprehensive challenges brought by the many vulnerable client groups currently actively seeking out reflexology, as well as provide students with a robust rationale for their practice.

Decades might pass before the complex mechanics of touch, and specifically the application of precise reflexology might be truly understood. The manner of research enquiry required to satisfy such an endeavour would require substantial financial funding. Presently within the medical world funding of that magnitude is simply not made available to study complementary therapies at such depth, perhaps precisely because there exists such little sound *acceptable* qualitative research to justify more expensive investigation. The question of how research funding is sourced also presents additional challenges for the complementary medicine world, given the percentage of medical research funded by pharmaceutical companies and those with corporate interests in medicine.

Future research then we can only hope will provide us with a deeper understanding of the precise mechanics of reflexology, and perhaps even go on to clarify definitions for standardising the reflexology *'foot map'*. Encouragingly more established modalities such as medical acupuncture have already gained some level of professional acknowledgement and respect from the scientific community. However, it is worth noting in the UK, acupuncture as 'treatment' option is currently only recognised officially by the National Health Service as being effective within a pain management context.

Reflexology has indeed many miles to go in terms of reaching even a similar level of acknowledgement, and until such a time is upon us, practitioners must strive to make good use of what has been already proven and demonstrated, both scientifically and academically, and continue to build on this fascinating work.

Psychoneuroimmunology is beginning to call together those previously fragmented medical, scientific, psychological and sociological disciplines. In the future this more complex multi-dimensional approach to understanding human health will undoubtedly require a far more complex holistic and kaleidoscopic form of research enquiry. An enquiry better suited to exploring the *multi-dimensional phenomenology of the reflexology package*. The future then indeed looks promising.

Practitioner responsibility

The responsibility of promoting safe practice extends not only to official bodies like the ASA or the professional reflexology associations. This attitude should also sit firmly at the core of every practitioner's rational for professional practice. Practitioners who wish to help protect and develop the future of reflexology must swiftly learn to communicate in a new and more informed therapeutic language.

The evidence incorporated in the relational reflexology practitioner's rationale for practice does not claim to cure or diagnose. The rationale is in fact firmly supported by a valid scientific hypothesis suggesting touch and reflexology can, within the context of a wider therapeutic environment, promote a lessening of perceived stress in clients and help to encourage self directed, autonomous change. Lessening of perceived stress potentially leads to fewer instances of stimulation occurring in the HPA axis. In turn this reduces the possibility of perturbations occurring in gonadotrophin levels, and menstrual and ovulatory patterns, therefore promoting the provision of the 'hospitable womb'.

How though do professional practitioners, in the face of such a lack of acceptable scientific research and fear, make a professional decision about whether it is correct to respond to the sub-fertility client asking to be supported? How do we marry for example, the qualitative experience of reflexology with the measurable and quantifiable experience of IVF? Here we turn to the subject of developing our own *inner supervisors* as holistic and complementary therapists, and learning to hone our personal ethical decision making processes.

Ethical decision making

The challenge in ethical decision making is to balance our real and perceived fears and concerns against our knowledge and experience, ideally arriving at a decision or a state of being where we feel comfortable in our ability to confidently meet the presenting needs of our client. A good rule when making an ethical decision is where no clear path is illuminated, one should take the path that causes least harm. Put simply, if you are unsure, do not proceed. ***Beneficence*** is an ethical principle most connected with applying therapeutic skills to help people. It relates to and might be defined as actions which are taken to benefit another. In complementary therapies the duty of beneficence must be considered together with its converse duty; that of ***non-maleficence,*** which is the concept well of ensuring no-one is hurt. This principle should ensure that any risks involved are proportionate to the benefits.

In essence the process of deciding if the challenge of this complex work is suitable for each practitioner will be an individual one. A decision made based on existing theoretical understanding, training and overall experience. It is the individual practitioner alone who must decide if they feel they are experienced or competent in the application of that information to attempt to meet the extensive needs of the potential sub-fertility or IVF client. Practitioners must develop their own *inner supervisors* if they are to practice ethically.

Continuing professional development

"A working knowledge of counselling can be a potent tool in drawing out the whole picture to help practitioners offer the best treatment" (March-Smith, 2005)

It would be wrong to pass through a chapter addressing the ethics of working in sub-fertility and supported ART work without taking some time to consider CPD and additional training. It is hoped as the practitioner fully absorbs and integrates the information presented in this book they will also become more aware of the importance of also considering additional training. Even a basic counselling skills course affords practitioner an awareness of how to build effective listening relationship, and how to offer active listening skills. Courses such as these often additionally explore safeguarding procedures and boundary issues. Developing these skills undoubtedly adds to the depth and effectiveness of any practitioner working with vulnerable client groups.

For practitioners to internally question if they possess the appropriate skills to meet the needs of a client is entirely ethical and appropriate. To use a useful analogy; a generically qualified counsellor might still think twice about engaging in a therapeutic relationship with a client experiencing post traumatic stress disorder. Without adequate specialised training the therapist, no matter how well meaning may not possess the appropriate skills set required to meet the specific needs of the client. In acknowledging this and in perhaps signposting the client to a more experienced or appropriately qualified practitioner is to work professionally and ethically. Engaging with sub-fertility clients requires the same dedication of focus upon the client needs. Where additional training might be required to ensure confidence and excellence of practice, it remains the practitioner's ethical responsibility to engage in that training.

Developing informed knowledge

It is essential that practitioners choosing to engage with sub-fertility clients or indeed any vulnerable client group are able to meet clients with an appropriate level of informed knowledge, in addition to a technical proficiency in the application of their therapeutic modality. Women undertaking fertility treatment are for the most part educated regarding their medical conditions. They understand what a FSH level is and might have been tracking their ovulation regularly. They talk in abbreviations of TTC (trying to conceive) and are very familiar with medical terminology. Sub-fertility clients may have been thinking, dreaming and reading about only pregnancy for many months and many will have done so in great detail.

Practitioners must be appropriately educated in order to provide clients with a safe therapeutic environment. The practitioner must know to reassure a client when she mentions feeling worried by the down-regulating nasal spray running down her throat during week two of an IVF protocol that doctors have compensated for this in the medication, and in fact it is a very common occurrence. If the practitioner panics because he or she doesn't know, then the client is likely to remain fearful also. Again, it remains the practitioner's ethical responsibility to engage in any required additional training, and to source any specialist reading material to better ensure a high level of proficiency in practice.

Practitioner self care

Any practitioner considering working with a client group associated with deep emotional strains should be aware of the impact this directly or indirectly might have on their own personal emotional health. It would be unprofessional and unrealistic not to acknowledge the emotional *baggage* complementary therapists deal with on a daily basis and with this particular client group comes many challenges.

An element of working ethically requires practitioners remain aware of their own personal needs and engage in appropriate self care. Not every client finds a happy ever after ending, and for those who do the road is often bumpy and filled with many pit-falls. Many reflexology and complementary therapy associations hold monthly support groups where therapists can learn from each other, share information and find support.

Professional practitioner supervision is discussed in more depth in chapter four.

Summary

Ask a G.P. their opinion on reflexology and most will either universally dismiss the modality as utter rubbish, or at best perhaps acknowledge the potential placebo effect and agree a foot rub can indeed be very relaxing! The medical world in general regards the benefits of reflexology poorly. Fundamentally this attitude exists for two reasons. Firstly practitioners are often poorly trained and cannot therefore communicate effectively a rational theoretical stance of practice, to either the public or to members of the medical community, and secondly, reflexology more often than not proves to be *inconclusive* when evaluated within quantitative methodology based research studies. The future reputation of reflexology therefore lies in the hands of every professional practitioner.

Developing a fuller understanding of precisely what defines a professional reflexology practice enables the practitioner to become more aware of the real and perceived boundaries and limitations in practice as well as helping to develop both personal and professional self awareness.

Developing a professional rationale for ethical practice can also help to clarify the relational reflexology practitioners acknowledgment of the various elements involved within the modality, and to consider how these individual dynamics might be working together to encourage positive therapeutic change in clients.

These are the ***real*** reflexology practitioner tools required to invoke and encourage real and lasting change in clients. These are also the tools required to practice reflexology responsibly, ethically and professionally.

CHAPTER THREE

WORKING WITH SUB-FERTILITY CLIENTS – A RATIONALE FOR PRACTICE

Understanding the fight or flight response

The fight or flight response is a primitive acute stress response linked to the sympathetic nervous system and controlled by the hypothalamus deep in the brain. There are more than 100 billion nerve cells responding to stimulus in the brain and forming an intricate network of communications. Some of the communications in the brain lead to conscious thought and action while others produce *autonomic responses* such as the fight or flight response. The aim of the fear response is to keep us safe and it is a vital part of our most basic human survival mechanisms.

The mind and fear trigger the fight or flight response in reaction to what the mind experiences as both *real and perceived* danger. When danger is registered the hypothalamus activates two systems; *the sympathetic nervous system and the adrenal-cortical system.* This physiologically linked autonomic response is characterised by an increase in heart rate and blood pressure, elevation of glucose levels in the blood, and redistribution of blood from the digestive tract to the muscles. The sympathetic nervous system uses nerve pathways to initiate reactions in the body, and the adrenal-cortical system uses the bloodstream. It is the combined effects of these two systems that make up the fight or flight response. The involvement of the sympathetic nervous system ensures the body speeds up and is ready to take action. The heart rate and blood pressure rise accordingly whilst signals are sent to muscles warning them to be alert. The stress hormones epinephrine (adrenaline) and norepinephrine (noradrenaline) are released into the bloodstream by the adrenal gland. Meanwhile the hypothalamus releases corticotropin-releasing factor (CRF) into the pituitary gland, activating the adrenal-cortical system. The pituitary gland in turn secretes the hormone ACTH (adrenocorticotropic hormone) which moves through the bloodstream, arriving at the adrenal cortex, where it activates the release of approximately 30 different hormones that help the body prepare to deal with the threat.

Stress responses are designed to *stand down* once the threat has passed. The opposing *relaxation response* occurs when the body is no longer in perceived danger and the functioning of the autonomic nervous system has returned to normal. The body thus moving from a state of physiological arousal to a state of physiological relaxation where blood pressure, heart rate, digestive functioning and hormonal levels all stabilise.

In today's modern world it is easy perhaps to imagine how persistent low level stress might be perceived and interpreted by the body as necessitating the activation of the fight or flight response. Consider for a moment the already anxious sub-fertility client who travels to work each day and sits for 8 hours fearful of attracting her superior's wrath, or the school teacher working late most nights trying to keep up with the paperwork. Real or perceived the body will react to the threat and the autonomic responses will be triggered. In times of low level and chronic stress to counteract the effect the *relaxation response* can be induced via an array of self help and supportive interventions. Supportive relational reflexology is but one such helpful intervention.

The hospitable womb - a rationale for practice

When considering the emotional and physical challenges faced by many sub-fertility clients it is easy to imagine why in this particular client group the fight or flight response might be on high alert. How might the body feel about the possibility of nurturing life when deep in the brain the perception is being processed as if the individual was being chased by a hungry lion or a similar type threat? The fear response makes no comparison between real and perceived fear. To the hypothalamus a bad tempered boss at work feels much the same as a hungry lion, and it will react accordingly.

Carl Rogers, a well know humanistic psychologist, proposed the existence of a *self–actualising tendency*. The self actualising tendency dictates all life possesses an innate drive to become everything it can be; to achieve its full potential. Self-actualising modern day human beings have learned to manipulate a woman's body into believing it is in a state of menopause only to be stimulated in the opposite direction to such a degree that multiple follicles and eggs are produced in the ovaries. That particular feat is balanced alongside assuring the lining of the womb develops sufficiently to host a returned fertilised embryo. Egg's are collected from ovaries microscopically and sparked into life by an embryologist using a microscope and a glass dish, before being returned to a woman's uterus. The IVF process is undoubtedly an astonishing scientific feat and a credit to the enquiring human mind. We are indeed fortunate to live in a society where such specialised clinical work is valued. A woman's inner drive to experience pregnancy and motherhood is absolutely deserving of such time, research and financial investment, and there are many women today who feel a huge debt of gratitude to specialist IVF and fertility units.

The writer is confident however even the most experienced consultants engaged in the field of IVF still scratch their heads from time to time and wonder why it is, even when top grade embryos are returned into a perfectly lined uterus, the generic success rate of IVF is around 26%? *(HFEA 2009)*

Research demonstrates success rates for frozen embryo transfers might be higher than those linked to conventional IVF protocols. It might be useful to reflect on the emotional mind-set of a woman who already knows she has potentially viable embryos available for transfer. How might this prior knowledge alter a women's perception of her chances of success?

Women in under-developed countries often live in poor conditions with little food, poor sanitation and little or no medical support. One thing is almost certain though. There are generally lots of babies around! What is perceived here in the West as an intensely stressful lifestyle is often but the norm for these women. Could this more normal frame of reference be dictating a more normally functioning HPA response? Admittedly we have the privilege of clean running water and central heating here in the West, but our stressful lifestyles and constant requirement to be ever productive and busy may well be leading us into disrespecting the innate autonomic systems deep within us. Systems designed by nature above all else to keep us safe.

> *"The fight of flight alarm reaction exists today for the same purpose evolution originally assigned to it; to enable us to survive. What has happened is that we have lost touch with the gut feeling designed to be out warning systems." (Mate, 2003).*

The self actualising tendency draws attention to the concept that life, given appropriate conditions to flourish, will often find a way to do so. Perhaps this concept might also be considered when attempting to appreciate why increasing numbers of women in the West are being diagnosed with non-specific sub-fertility and how this concept might also be impacting on IVF success rates? After all, there are many animals on our planet instinctively drawn to finding a safe place to nest before pro-creation occurs. Why would human beings be any different?

The concept of stress in our modern world has become somewhat lost and diluted and its consequences morphed to such a degree that dealing well with stress has almost become a badge of honour. Viewed as a sign of advanced coping mechanisms and an ability to successfully juggle all of life's complicated demands. In reality the principles of human homeostasis demonstrates quite clearly that for every *effect* there also exists a *counter effect*. Where high and sustained levels of stress exist in the human individual then perturbations across the wider endocrine system can also develop.

"Reproduction is one of the strongest of biological reflexes – just ask a salmon leaping upstream to spawn or male of various species risking life and limb for access to females, or any adolescent with that crazed steroid look. But when it comes to the pirouettes and filigrees of sexuality, stress can wreak havoc with subtleties." (Sapolsky, 2004).

Why relational reflexology to support sub-fertility clients?

Supportive relational reflexology, delivered by well trained and ethically driven practitioners, can provide sub-fertility clients with the perfect complementary therapeutic modality in which both body and mind-set can be encouraged towards achieving more regular states of the *relaxation state*, therefore promoting in women provision of 'the hospitable womb'.

Women's words on relational reflexology supporting sub-fertility

"(Reflexology) kept in my mind good health"

"Sessions have the ability to last a lifetime and extend far beyond the feet".

"(Reflexology) gave me the ability to put some perspective to what I was going through, to make sure I didn't allow it to take over my life completely"

"Physically I felt after each consultation that I was completely relaxed"

"I was mentally and physically prepared".

"(The therapist) truly empathised"

"(Reflexology) helped me to be more positive and I felt less stressed"

"After each appointment I felt refreshed and relaxed"

"Physically, my menstrual cycle started to change"

"Trying to have a family is all consuming and it can be hard to see anything outside that when you are stuck in the middle of it – (reflexology) managed to achieve that".

"I was better able to deal with my pain levels and felt emotionally stronger"

"I remember (the therapist) very delicately asking if I had anything else I was working on at the time. This jump started me to focus on other new projects which again helped me have a bit more control"

"To be understood as a person, rather than counted as an unwanted statistic makes every difference"

"I wish every woman battling fertility issues could be lucky enough to benefit from such therapy"

"(The therapist) understood me!!"

"(Reflexology) made me feel that I was doing all that I could possible do to improve our chances of conceiving. This was hugely empowering when I felt like I had little control over our future"

"I found the hour long sessions provided intense relaxation and it would lead to a better night's sleep"

A multi-dimensional modality

Reflexology seems to have morphed into a modern day complementary modality wearing many overcoats. Presently within our industry training can be accessed in (to name but a few) clinical reflexology; zone reflexology; vertical reflexology; meridian reflexology; gentle touch reflexology and more recently, a drastically diluted variation, principally practiced by beauty therapists. Regardless of the personal theoretical orientation of the practitioner, to the uninitiated reflexology might be most simply described as specific and applied stimulation of pressure to an extremity. In a Department of Health document aimed at primary care groups, reflexology is described as:

'the application of pressure to the hands and feet to promote well-being.' (Tiran & Mackereth, 2011)

Whilst we do not yet as a profession fully understand the precise mechanics of action relating to reflexology, we do know there exists a wealth of anecdotal evidence supporting its use across a wide range of conditions, in addition to a slowly growing body of *acceptable* scientifically recorded evidence.

It is not the writer's intention to discuss this vast subject here or to focus upon a lack of general consensus existing within the profession relating to basic principles and theoretical orientation. Rather the intention is simply *to acknowledge the generally accepted, physiologically relaxing and de-stressing state of being induced in many clients who receive reflexology as a specific pressure therapy.* In relational reflexology theoretical focus leans towards developing an appreciation of the commonalities existing within the reflexology package, regardless of the form or variation practiced by the individual practitioner.

Understanding more fully the potential multi-dimensional aspects of the reflexology package, and how the therefore the modality might be benefiting the sub-fertility group, requires a more detailed exploration of what might be happening within the confines of the reflexology practitioners consulting room.

Psychoneuroimmunoendocrinology

Psychoneuroimmunoendocrinology (PNI) is a relatively modern branch of scientific study which can be defined as an intention to investigate and better understand interactions between human psychological processes and that of the nervous and immune systems.

The main emphasis and drive in PNI therefore is to portray that complex biological systems are in essence integrated systems, and so the field focuses on studying the relationship between the components, rather than individually selected components.

PNI considers connections between the brain and immune system, and how stress and the mind can influence the body and vice versa. A fascinating field of research for holistic practitioner, PNI potentially offers a measure of validity to the holistic approach. The field supports the holistic and integrative rationale for practice stating the human mind and body are undoubtedly intertwined and connected, and therefore the experiences and perceptions of the individual can indeed directly affect wider physiological functions.

What defines stress?

Stress is a "complicated cascade of physical and biochemical responses to powerful emotional stimuli." (Mate, 2003)

The experience of stress can be defined as consisting of three components. Initially there is the physical or emotional (real or perceived) event interpreted as threatening to the individual *(the stress stimulus).* Secondly there is the processing system which interprets experiences and meaning *(the brain),* and finally the stress response itself, consisting of both *psychological and behavioural reactions and adjustments.* (Mate, 2003). The experience of stress and exactly how the individual reacts to a particular stressor is entirely unique.

"Stress is fundamentally a response to contextual change. Context is conceptualised in terms of social factors, the influence of other life forms, the non-living aspects of the environment and the characteristics of the individual. (Daruna, 2012).

Our unique physiological and psychological make-up therefore dictates our individual reactions and responses to stress. Defining and measuring precisely how stress affects the body, given our unique individual responses, presents a complex challenge for modern day medicine.

"The medical approach to health and illness continues to suppose that the body and mind are separable from each other and from the milieu in which they exist. Compounding that mistake is definition of stress that is narrow and simplistic." (Mate 2003).

Stress in the modern world

Modern woman certainly has her work cut out. What has been gained over a century in terms of freedom and equality has also led to the wide spread use of synthetic female contraception and an increase in Western women waiting until their thirties to start a family. By the time many women do decide to start a family many are already engaged in stressful careers and jobs. Women today have the responsibility of bills to pay and the rush hour to endure. Holidays are limited to four or five weeks per year and many sub-fertility clients report working on the laptop to meet deadlines and stay ahead of the workload, long after the working day has ended.

The days of a woman washing on a Monday, cleaning windows on a Tuesday and changing beds on a Wednesday are long gone and forgotten. Our Grandmother's and Great-Grandmothers stressors were real enough. Those stressors however might be defined as a shared and acknowledged wider society experience. Everybody had too little in those days, bar a few who 'lived on the hill' in elevated position and wealth! Our modern day stresses are much more silent and internal.

The stressors we experience today may well be shared experiences, but they are generally not commonly acknowledged, nor is it perceived often as wise to admit to we're not coping well with stress. The result? In today's modern busy world it has become increasingly common for individuals to become detached from their own innate physiological *felt sense.* In other words their ability to read the internal signals the body sends. Insomnia, dizziness, chest tightness, feeling nauseous, churning in the stomach, neck tension and even physical shaking, can all be signs of emotional distress (in fact taken to the extreme, panic attacks can often display many of the above symptoms), but how many people ignore warning signs such as these? The pressures of modern life with our determination to do well and achieve, and our personal inner drives to find acceptance and a perfect piece of happiness have unfortunately resulted in increasing levels of disassociation from our true emotional states.

Scientists spend time forcing rats, mice and monkeys into construed situations so they might attempt to measure the physiological and psychological effects of stress. Really we only need to look at human behaviour in our modern world to roughly gauge the effects of stress. It doesn't look so good. It seems modern day human beings are dealing with excessive pressure at every turn. Pressure to be accepted, pressure to succeed, pressure to hit deadlines and pay bills, pressure to simply survive! The internal pressures we place upon ourselves in terms of how we are perceived by family, friends and our wider society, and indeed the pressures we are forced to react to daily are only a reflection of the busy, competitive, driven societies we now live in.

Gabor Mate is entirely correct when he states we overly simplify the concept of stress. Our profit driven materialistic and often highly judgmental societies encourage us not to present ourselves in any way as tired, weak, fearful, or indecisive. We are encouraged instead to plough on regardless and just deal with our stress quietly. In doing so we often ignore our true feelings and levels of personal exhaustion. Humans have become in fact the only creatures on this beautiful blue planet who don't stop to snooze in the mid-day sun and admire the view. Instead we are busy meeting deadlines, trying to avoid the boss and somehow fit in the weekly shop! Being cognitively smart and high functioning doesn't mean though our emotions don't count.

> *"Repression – disassociating emotions from awareness and relegating them to the unconscious realm – disorganizes and confuses our physiological defenses."* (Mate, 2003).

Better connecting to our inner *felt sense* can help us to recognize and acknowledge our emotional reactions, giving voice to them and helping to reduce the effect of stress before they begin to cascade further inwards. It is also worth remembering, particularly in the case of the sub-fertility client, that stress responses are reactive to perceived fear, as well real life threats.

> *"The stress-response can be mobilized not only in response to physical or psychological insults, but also in expectation of them – a physiological system activated not only by all sorts of physical disasters but by just thinking about them as well." (Sapolsky, 2004).*

The very moment a woman perceives there might be a problem with her fertility, that thought, that fear, only serves to compound the physiological problem. Better appreciating then our real emotional state and learning to give voice to our feelings can help us to live more authentic lives. It is this *authenticity* in experiencing that the body is able to register as entirely normal and baseline, and it is from this place bodily functions are able to maintain a more natural state of homeostasis.

Our Grandmothers undoubtedly worked hard and often struggled through great adversity but their experiences were shared and voiced as universally common place. Today women dealing with sub-fertility issues suffer alone in silence, often afraid to speak their truth. Life is complex and the stressors are multiple!

Stress and Pregnancy

Studies examining the influence psychoneuroendocrine processes might have on foetal development and health demonstrate both cardiovascular and neuroendocrine responses to stressors are attenuated during human pregnancy and that increased cardiovascular reactivity is associated with: *"shorter gestation, lower birth weight, increased risk of preeclampia and vulnerability for postpartum depression."* (Christian, 2012).

Researchers (Wadhwa, 2005) believe maternal stress responses may indeed have life-long effects on off-spring health and that: *"maternal environment exerts significant influence on foetal neurodevelopmental processes related to recognition, memory and habituation."* Research (Culhane, Rauh, Farley-McCollum, Hogan, Agnew, & Wadhwa, 2001) looking at maternal psychosocial stress its influence on the development of reproductive tract infections amongst a large group of socially disadvantaged women found; *"stress related endocrine processes modulate immune function in the context of reproductive tract infection and inflammation."* Studies have also demonstrated that interventions such as guided imagery, yoga and relaxation (DiPietro, Mendelson, Williams, & Costigan, 2011); (Urich, Simons, Losito, Fiorito, Miles, & Zelson, 1991); (Beddoe, Paul Yang, Kennedy, Weiss, & Lee, 2009); *(Beddoe & Lee, 2008)* can be effective in reducing maternal heart rate and subjective feelings of stress.

Stress and sub-fertility

In normally responding individuals the brain releases GnRH (gonadotrophin releasing hormone), which stimulates the pituitary to release LH (luteinizing hormone) and FHS (follicle stimulating hormone). Luteinizing hormone stimulates the ovaries to synthesise estrogen and the testes to release testosterone. The activation of FSH in women stimulates the ovaries to release eggs, and in men stimulates sperm production.

Stress has been demonstrated to elevate levels of adrenocorticotropic hormone (ACTH) and cortisol in the blood and researchers believe these increases may; *"at least temporarily amplify the effects of the pituitary-adrenal axis on other tissues."* (Daruna, 2012). Because the hypothalamus is in two-way communication with the brain centre that process emotions, *"it is through the HPA axis that emotions exert their most direct effects on the immune system and on other organs."* (Mate, 2003).

Indeed stress has been demonstrated as activating the hypothalmic-pituitary-adrenal (HPA) axis in turn inhibits gonadotrophin-releasing hormone (Gn-RH) release, possibly through the effects of opioid peptides. Inhibition of Gn-RH release leads to decreased luteinizing hormone (LH) and follicle-stimulating hormone (FSH) levels in the circulation and ultimately reduced estradiol in females and testosterone in males. *"Thus psychosocial stress appears to cause the decrease of gonadal steroids."* (Daruna, 2012).

The HPA axis and the reproductive system demonstrate a complex relationship. CRH and cortisol receptors are *"abundant in the endometrium, myometrium, and the ovaries."* (Demyttenaere, Nijs, Evers-Keibooms, & Koninckx, 1994). Stress can also inhibit progesterone levels which can disrupt the maturation of the uterine walls. The release of prolactin during times of stress can further interfere with the activity of progesterone, making any fertilised egg *"much less likely to implant normally"*. (Sapolsky, 2004).

In a study published in the 'Canadian Journal of Diagnosis' (Prior, 1997) found that *"subtle hormonal disruption can even occur amongst women who report regular periods and no symptoms"*, the study also demonstrated anovulation problems in women *"are caused by adaptations to life cycle, changes in weight, psychosocial stresses, excessive exercise or illness."* Indeed experts believe the hormones related to female reproduction to be *"exquisitely sensitive to women's psychological states and to the stresses in their lives."* (Mate, 2003).

When considering the emotional stresses and challenges faced by many modern women, and in further acknowledging that feelings of stress are often compounded by the fear of infertility, it is then perhaps easy to imagine why innate evolutionary biological mechanisms might try to prevent pregnancy.

Given the already proven effects of stress on both fetal development and maternal health, it seems perhaps logical that complex systems within the body might be triggered into setting into action a *biological defense mechanism* which might prevent conception occurring in the first instance. An evolutionary defense mechanism ultimately designed to protect the life energy of the host organism, the mother.

Stress and IVF

One of the main difficulties in evaluating the success rate of IVF is establishing the particular factors which make a real difference. Experts such as Robert Sapolsky *(2004),* a professor of biology and neurology at Stanford University, believe the *'stressfulness'* of IVF procedures contribute to the low success rates. Interestingly, IVF patients with functional disorders of the HPA axis often demonstrate higher stress-scores than women where sub-fertility is associated with anatomical problems (tube obstruction, malformations of the reproductive organs). It has also been demonstrated that stress and anxiety are very common in sub-fertility patients, especially those undergoing IVF (Salvatore, Gariboldi, Offidani, Coppola, Amore, & Maggini, 2001).

Some IVF studies have demonstrated that the chance to conceive and to bring the pregnancy to a good end is smaller if the patient reports more stress or anxiety at the onset of therapy (Demyttenaere, Nijs, Evers-Keibooms, & Koninckx, 1994). In 2008 (Manheimer, Zhang, & Udoff, 2008) provided an overview of the effect of acupuncture on IVF, comparing the results of seven different trials, including 1366 women. Results overall demonstrate the application of acupuncture immediately before and after embryo transfer improves rates of pregnancy and live birth among women undergoing IVF.

Another small research study (Balk, Catov, Horn, Gecsi, & Wakim, 2009) specifically looked at the relationship between perceived stress, acupuncture, and pregnancy in IVF patients. In this study the mechanism of acupuncture was not specifically studied. Rather the research attempted to establish if *perceived* stress factored in IVF success rates. The study utilised a 10-item stress questionnaire to establish patients stress levels before and during embryo transfer; concluding; *"The acupuncture regimen was associated with less stress both before and after embryo transfer and it possibly improved pregnancy rates. Lower perceived stress at the time of embryo transfer may play a role in an improved pregnancy rate".*

Reflexology and stress

Reflexology has gained public recognition for helping to reduce feelings of stress in clients. Why might that be? Peter Mackereth believes the reflexology exchange may be impacting clients multi-dimensionally;

> *"Emotional reactions to a series of treatments are not uncommon in bodywork, and the nurturing use of touch and support and acceptance that evolve in the therapeutic relationship may tacitly give permission for this." (Tiran & Mackereth, 2011).*

With Mackereth additionally stating:

> *"Therapists using touch in the form of reflexology may not consciously be within a psychodynamic contract, but the effect on self-image is likely to have some potency and subsequent health benefits."*

These statements clearly highlight touch, self-image, support, acceptance and the therapeutic relationship as important elements to be considered when attempting to account for some of the collective phenomenological reactions clients can report. Supporting the concept of reflexology promoting stress reduction specifically, Mackereth believes the reflexology package might be assisting in the release of endorphins (and a) reduction in cortisol and other stress hormones.

In a Korean study (Jang & Kim, 2009) researchers examined the effects self-foot massage in middle aged menopausal women, concluding; *"Reflexology may be an effective nursing intervention in reducing perceived stress, fatigue and blood circulation."* Another study (Quattrin, et al., 2006) examined the effectiveness of reflexology in reducing anxiety among hospitalized cancer patients, concluding reflexology, in combination with other treatments, *"can help (patients) feel better and also cope with their disease."*

Touch

For the purpose of this section the word touch can be defined within a therapeutic context as:

> *"that which is not intended to stimulate or elicit sexual feelings, nor is it regarded culturally as sexual". Uphoff (Haugh & Paul, 2008).*

In ancient Shamanic healing traditions the application of touch was often utilised. We know that acupressure was practiced in China thousands years ago and that the Persians, Egyptians, Greeks and Romans all consulted healer priests throughout the reign of their respective civilizations, with touch as an integral element of many of these healing encounters.

Human beings communicate through touch on many different levels. A more casual form of touch might involve simply a handshake or a reassuring pat on the arm. The manner in which we touch our partners or children might be more focused and applied with more intention and care. Touch has the ability to communicate our feelings without words. Consider for a moment a parent crossing a busy road with a young child. As the adult quietly squeezes the child's hand more firmly, the parent is communicating their intention clearly through the medium of touch, and a child will often become aware of the message implied; be safe and hang on tight!

Scientific research provides us with a better understanding of the beneficial effects of touch to the human body. The skin is the largest organ in the human body and loaded with receptors associated with touch, pain, temperature and pressure;

> *"Touch is an important part of being human, a way in which our consciousness is redrawn into our physical being and our very existence confirmed."* (Jourard, 1966)

Research supporting the application of touch therapeutically, such as carried out by (DeAngelis & Mwakalyelye, 1995) concluded for example, babies who were stroked regularly were healthier and thrived better than those babies receiving no touch. The study interestingly also concluded mothers who received massage were "*less depressed and anxious*" than those who received only relaxation training.

Similarly, an Australian study reviewing the effectiveness of complementary therapies for anxiety in both children and adolescents showed that massage has "*immediate and short-term effects on anxiety*" (Paslow, Morgan, Allan, Jorm, O'Donnell, & Purcell, 2007). Another study (Birk, 2000) looked at the effectiveness of massage therapy alone and in combination with other complementary therapies in HIV patients. The study demonstrated that "*Massage combined with stress management favorably alters health perceptions.*

Touch as a physiological interaction has been clinically proven to aid the release of endorphins as well as the neuropeptides, serotonin and dopamine. When released into the bloodstream these chemicals serve to counteract and suppress the effects of adrenal stress hormones such as cortisone and adrenaline (Field, Hernandez-Reif, & Diego, 2005). From a psychological perspective appropriate touch is viewed positively and widely acknowledged as an important element of many human interactions. Appropriate touch is viewed for example as absolutely necessary to children both psychologically and developmentally, and touch has been identified in many studies as promoting reassurance and affirmation of existence. Indeed researchers have found touch could be:

> *"identified as having the potential to trigger a catharsis, to be a catalyst for meaningful change, to provide a corrective emotional experience." (Williams, Clarke, & Gibson, 2011).*

Therapeutic Touch

Historically, the healing modality of Therapeutic Touch was pioneered by Delores Kreiger, a Professor of Nursing at New York University, and is widely taught across both the USA and Canada and considered as a natural extension of nursing skills. Therapeutic touch can be distinguished from most other bio-energetic therapies because the modality has been demonstrated to be effective after extensive, empirical investigation (Graham, 1999).

Therapeutic Touch can be carried out using either physical or non-physical contact. In essence the practitioner is attempting to focus her attention inwards to achieve a relaxed and focused state in which she can make an *assessment* of a patient's energetic body field. The practitioner attempts to achieve this by developing an awareness of sensations in her own hands and wider body. The patients affected area is then balanced using colour imagery as a focus for directing healing energies, for example, red to warm and stimulate an area; blue to cool or sedate and yellow to energise. When the practitioner becomes aware of the patients energetic body field feeling more balanced the healing session is considered complete. Ask many experienced reflexologists to describe their intention and intuition relating to their reflexology practice and many similarly describe a feeling of *intuitively* understanding when the feet feel more balanced, with many practitioners re-working areas of the feet which seem to be calling for additional attention.

A therapeutic relationship

There are then perhaps some obvious similarities existing between energetic modalities such as therapeutic touch and pressure modalities such as reflexology. Practitioners of TT interestingly also seem to be demonstrating an *attentiveness* within their modality dedicated towards patient experience. In client focused talking therapies, such as person-centred counselling, this interaction between two human beings, both focused on the experiencing of the client, is considered to be of paramount importance, and this *focused interaction* forms an equally integral part of working relationally as a professional reflexologist.

Reflexology practitioners are often adept at focusing on the physical feel of the feet and body, and of focusing their attention and energy towards their client. In relational reflexology the same focus of attention is required, however practitioners are encouraged to widen their viewpoint and develop a deeper appreciation of the dynamic nature of human exchanges, and what might define a therapeutic encounter.

Supporting the concept of emotional movement as a result of holistic treatments, Mitchell and Cormack *(1998)* state; *"psychological or interpersonal processes inevitably form part of all treatment encounters."* Whilst Mackereth *(2011)* referring to reflexology specifically believes physiological changes can occur as a consequence of psychological processes and given the complexity of the reflexology package these are likely to be *"working in synergy"*, additionally stating (reflexology) can provide a space for *"psychological support and nurturing of the body."*

"the psychological impact of treatment cannot be disregarded and may, indeed, play a fundamental role in the mechanism of action."(Tiran, 2011)

Research carried out for Christie NHS Foundation, Manchester, (Makereth, Booth, Hillier, & Caress, 2009) exploring the nature of the interaction between clients and complementary therapists. The results revealed that *"reflexology provided opportunities for 48 out of the 50 participants to share worries and concerns".*

The study further concluded that reflexology appeared to have created a space for patients to talk about their worries and concerns and to receive advice and support from the nurse therapists. This research seems to suggest that from the client's perspective some therapeutic benefit is being derived from the holistic environment, and clients often feel they can talk freely to their reflexology practitioners. The research also demonstrated, via the analysis of taped transcripts of reflexology treatments, that there were numerous examples of client originated reflexology related enquiries occurring during treatments, leading to further *"disclosures of worries and concerns."* Similarly (Gambles, Crooke, & Wilkinson, 2002) used semi structured questionnaires to uncover the existential benefits of reflexology treatments from the client's perspective and the evidence seemed to add to the suggestion that reflexology, far from solely being a physiologically stimulating pressure therapy, also contains an element identified very clearly as *relational* in essence:

"Being able to discuss my illness with caring and friendly staff"

"I just talked which was also very helpful"

"I had so much on my mind"

"The (therapist) was so helpful and caring"

"She helped me with advice"

Research providing us with a valid analysis of the results of specifically blending, for example, the two modalities of reflexology and counselling is still in its infancy. A small quantitative research project (Trousdell & Uphoff-Chmielnic, 1997) looking at the efficiency of delivering reflexology and person-centred counselling 'concomitantly' over the same time period indicated:

"Client's receiving both therapies moved to significantly more positive psychological posture and physical well-being within a shorter time than expected."

Wider professional promotion championing the benefits of developing a deeper appreciation of the nature of the therapeutic relationship; and indeed how the professional practitioner's reflexology session might be enhanced, or a client even ethically protected as a result of increased knowledge, could only improve professional standards within our industry. Long term, increased awareness might also be the single defining factor which brings into focus a more definite professional line between spa and beauty type reflexology treatments, and those carried out by well trained and educated practitioners engaging with diagnosed, clinical conditions and offering supportive reflexology to more vulnerable client groups.

Taking control – the existential benefit for clients

The relational reflexology relationship, supported by appropriate knowledge can also be utilised to encourage better nutritional self care, as well as promoting more regular instances of focused relaxation extending beyond the confines of supportive reflexology sessions. Interventions of this nature can be utilised to encourage clients to make more time for self care and perhaps restructure life commitments where possible. This can help to promote feelings of being more in control, pro-active and calm, thus reducing the potential of prolonged fight of flight responses.

Well informed practitioners utilising a developed and accurate knowledge of anatomy and physiology, for example, might be appropriately viewed as educating and engaging the client in the workings of her own body, potentially helping the client to connect more fully to her experience.

Collaborative work can facilitate huge changes, whether that advice relates to education, effective sign posting, dietary advice or teaching a client a relaxing deep breathing technique. Practical well informed guidance can be utilised both ethically and productively.

Promoting existential thinking

Existentialism in a broader sense might be defined as a philosophy which centres upon the analysis of human existence. Existentialism is primarily concerned with developing the self and a meaning for life through individual free will, choice, and personal responsibility. Pure existential thought promotes the concept that an individual should be responsible for themselves, without the help of laws, ethnic rules, or traditions. Existential thinking therefore often focuses on:

Self-awareness and more authentic living - People often avoid listening to themselves and their real needs and desires and this can sometimes results in painful inner conflicts, unhappiness, and feelings of powerlessness. Thinking more existentially, the individual can find his inner voice and guidance and become more aware and authentic in making choices.

Responsibility for decisions - Existential thinking can help individuals to become more aware of their freedom, choices, and the potential consequences of their actions. This type of thinking can help people develop a better sense of how they are 'authors' of their experiencing.

Developing personal meaning - Existential thinking can help individuals to uncover personal meaning and truths in their lives (including meaning from painful experiences) through personal reflection. Existential thinkers believe both emptiness and meaninglessness in life can lead to feelings of despair.

Coping with anxiety - Existential thinking can help individuals examine the roots of some of their anxieties and learn how to better cope with them.

Living in the present moment - Existential thinking helps an individual to understand how to live in the moment, and that everything changes. Life can often then be experienced more authentically, in the here and now, more present in each moment.

The benefit of promoting existential thinking is that it can help clients to choose from different ways of living and experiencing, as well as promoting free will. Relational reflexology practitioners are in a position to promote more existential choice in their clients primarily through encouragement and education.

Consider for a moment the PCOS client, recently diagnosed with a disorder closely linked to insulin resistance. Administering reflexology to support this condition without exploring and promoting with the client the benefits of adopting a type II diabetic eating pattern might seem an opportunity missed to promote positive change. Helping clients to understand why it would be beneficial to the endocrine system and long-term well-being and therefore promoting choice, the well informed complementary therapist is supporting her client as she ideally becomes more pro-active and engaged in her own healthcare. Benefiting not only the physical body, but also promoting more helpful thinking patterns.

Setting clients small tasks or SMART (small measurable, attainable, realistic and time-limited) goals to complete between sessions can prove invaluable in helping clients to feel more engaged and pro-active in their journey. Emotional stressful conditions such as sub-fertility which perhaps carry previous long-term historical disappointment mean it can be easy for clients to slip into negative, automatic patterns of thinking. A more balanced form of thinking is more likely to occur when the mind is occupied with pro-active, helpful activities. These activities are utilised primarily to promote client-centred time in the day and focus on client self care. This topic is discussed in more detail in chapter five.

Summary

The core rationale for engaging in relational reflexologist with sub-fertility clients centres firmly around the concept of promoting the 'hospitable womb' in women through attempting to reduce frequent activation of the HPA axis in the body. The rationale is supported by scientific principles of psychoneuroimmunology (PNI) and accepted connections between the mind, stress and the body's physiological functions.

Developing a professional rationale for practice, through better understanding our own practice can help to ensure sound professional ethics and boundaries exist in the work we engage in.

It is essential practitioners are able to explain and justify their stance and rationale of practice so to be more accepted and integrated as complementary practitioners. Developing an appreciation for the various elements existing within the confines of the reflexology exchange also means practitioners are better able to begin to appreciate the *totality* of what supportive relational reflexology can offer to clients. The modality, practiced within the confines of a supportive relationship can provide clients with a holistic experience perhaps well equipped to support the unique oneness of a client; a modality able to embrace and appreciate the individuality of the unique individual, as well as acknowledge the commonly shared biologically and physiologically innate.

CHAPTER FOUR

THE THERAPEUTIC RELATIONSHIP – RELATIONAL DEPTH IN REFLEXOLOGY

"Part of being compassionate and present in therapeutic work is to recognise the honour of witnessing another who is experiencing emotional vulnerability" (Tiran & Mackereth, 2011)

The emotional impact of sub-fertility

"Everywhere I go I feel like I'm being stalked by pregnant women. It just seems so unfair." This statement is fairly representative of the feelings of many women who enter a therapy room looking for support with sub-fertility. The statement perhaps best reflects the duality of a woman's experience emotionally. Initially we're drawn to almost a fixation with pregnancy; to the extent that everywhere the woman turns she can see pregnancy in others. The second part of the statement perhaps simply expresses the deep sadness and grief like feelings often experienced by these women. Indeed grief, sadness, anger, frustration, anxiety and fear are all familiar emotions for the sub-fertility client.

Women sometimes talk of their deep sadness when friends become pregnant, and then their later feelings of shame because they know deep inside they feel envious. Some women find the sight of a pregnant woman difficult to endure, whilst for others it is the sight of a mother pushing her pram. Siblings, relations, friends, workmates and even hardly known acquaintances all seem to be able to pro-create easily enough without assistance and irritatingly some even go on to do it twice! Women come to know their bodies intimately charting basal temperatures and testing for ovulation, yet often lose faith in their bodies completely. Women recount tails of engaging robotically with their partners and husbands, and talk of how fertility problems have damaged their sex life and feelings of intimacy and closeness. The dreaded arrival of the menstrual bleed is simply a reminder of how they have failed again, each month, each failure only adding to their deep sub-conscious fear that they will never become pregnant.

Women dealing with sub-fertility can exist in a state of pretending to be happy on the surface whilst experiencing deep pain on the inside. Friends and family smile supportively and make noises of optimism and bright futures. Comments like 'you just need to relax' or 'have a holiday' are well meant and common place, yet all the while the women alone with their fears are screaming inside, tortured by a never-ending longing to have a baby.

It might take the average woman between two and three years of trying to conceive naturally before she is referred to a specialist unit. The sub-fertility journey can take an enormous toll both physically and emotionally.

The emotional impact of IVF

It is important to remember that for most women undergoing IVF being referred to a specialist fertility unit is but the latest stop on a very long journey. Initially, most women feel only relief when an IVF referral letter arrives. Finally they will see the doctors who really know what they're doing! Then arrives the day of the first appointment and no matter how well trained and welcoming the unit staff are, no matter how inviting the environment, the moment a woman is given the date schedule for her IVF protocol, and she becomes aware of what lies ahead of her fear and panic often set in.

No matter how astonishing the science of IVF might be the reality of the protocol for most women might be best described as negotiating a path of hurdles. One cannot move forward to the next phase of treatment until X, Y or Z has been achieved, and at all times there is a worry the protocol might be abandoned if the woman does not respond accordingly. If the protocol is completed through to the egg collection phase attention turns to the concern of how many eggs will be retrieved successfully. Of those eggs how many will fertilise successfully and will they be good enough grade embryos?

Post embryo transfer, a woman waits and tries hard not to agonise over the next ten days until either a menstrual bleed occurs spontaneously, or a test confirms either a pregnancy or a failed cycle. It is easy to imagine how a woman might find this entire process deeply stressful.

It would clearly be entirely unprofessional to attempt any variety of therapeutic work with this client group without a first having a deep respect and understanding of how sub-fertility has impacted across the lives of each woman. The sub-fertility journey is massively disempowering for women. It is journey in which a woman can lose not only connection and trust with her body, but also with hope and her future. Both mind and body equally challenged.

Women's words on sub-fertility

"I thought (pregnancy) would never happen""

I am alone in it all"

"Constant bleeding and hormonal irregularity meant my body felt completely alien to me"

"I'd become a shadow of the person I used to be"

"You try to remain positive and happy but it hurts, and you start to wonder what you've done wrong to deserve such a harsh punishment"

"After 3 unsuccessful IVF attempts we were left devastated"

"Every advert seems to be baby stuff: every soap (on tv) has an unwanted pregnancy story!"

"Hubby tries to be supportive but each month when I get upset he tells me 'I told you not to get your hopes up!' How can you remain positive and upbeat and not hope each month?"

"I felt it was all my fault"

"Simple day to day tasks were crushing. Walking round the supermarket through aisles of babies in prams, or expectant mothers tenderly rubbing their growning bumps made me want to stay at home and hide from the world"

"Everything seemed to come back to one thought; will I have another baby?"

"I realised how stressed and deflated I had become as a result of the repeated failures".

Client disclosure - an elephant in the room

In recent years it would be fair to say two distinctly different forms of reflexology have developed. Increased recognition of the modality within the media and general public means reflexology is now commonly found as a treatment option within many beauty salons and spas. This form of reflexology is often, but not exclusively, carried out by beauty therapists and an increasing number of practitioners with a duel interest in beauty and holistic work.

Conversely there exists a group of more traditionally minded practitioners, perhaps more familiar in encountering clients diagnosed with specific clinical conditions and disorders. Practitioners often go on to develop their own personal style of practice, with some leaning towards adopting a more clinical, physiological rationale for their work, whilst others will prefer to focus on providing a calming spa type ambience and third group will be drawn towards developing a more integrative, relational approach.

Few practitioners, regardless of their form of practice would deny client disclosures take place regularly within complementary therapy practices. The stance of the various professional bodies leans towards encouraging external referral to an appropriately qualified counsellor when it becomes apparent a client is dealing with emotional issues. Safe practice is primarily promoted by discouraging reflexologists from interacting verbally with clients outside of the consultation period, guiding towards avoiding emotional exchanges wherever possible. Professional boundaries are of course rightly in place to prevent practitioners who do not possess appropriate training, knowledge or expertise from stepping outside of their professional competency. These boundaries can seem relatively clear and easy to follow on paper however setting realistic boundaries within a working reflexology practice can often be a little more challenging.

It would perhaps be rather naive to imagine a world where women seeking reflexology to support their sub-fertility issues were able to leave their emotions conveniently at the practitioner's front door. It might also be a little naive to imagine practitioners who were initially drawn to training in a healing modality, such as reflexology, might somehow find it relatively easy to turn a blind eye to potential emotional distress in a client.

In accepting a more realistic definition of the nature of human exchanges, and in order for best practice to flourish, practitioners must take responsibility for their own personal and professional development, through actively widening their professional skills set and acknowledging the responsibility of working with sub-fertility clients. Practitioners must in essence develop their own inner supervisors and be ready to judge themselves as competent to practice with emotionally vulnerable client groups.

Encouragingly often the clearest and easiest ethically boundaries to maintain professionally are those which emanate from the individual practitioner; when something feels right or wrong it is often easier to make a clear choice. The well developed practitioner who has engaged in appropriate further training and thus assured herself she is ready to take on the task of engaging with an emotionally vulnerable client is a practitioner who is working authentically, ethically and effectively. Clearly the initial training pathway of the practitioner should in no way prevent professional development, however it is strongly recommended that only those practitioners who are open to acknowledging the potential emotional vulnerability of the sub-fertility group, and choose to engage in appropriate steps to ensure excellence and competence in their practice, should consider engaging in this type of work.

Going deeper in reflexology - seeing past the feet

Providing clients with a safe and supportive therapeutic space in which to disclose information might appropriately be considered as nurturing and respecting the human mind and emotions, in addition to the physiological body we're so used to dealing with as modern practitioners of reflexology.

"The main thrust in alternative, or complementary, therapy training has been on healing. Body and soul are fully acknowledged; yet the mind seems, somewhat surprisingly for holistic workers, to have taken a back seat" (March-Smith, 2005).

A part of working holistically relates to valuing and considering individual client phenomenology as multi-dimensional in essence. As we've already discussed, within a relational reflexology context it can be helpful to place value on the individual elements collectively forming a modern day reflexology session. The nature and power held within the therapeutic relationship is one such vitally important element.

The term therapeutic relationship might also be called a helping or working alliance. The term is often used to describe the working relationship between any health-care professional and a client or patient. A great deal of research has been undertaken in the field of counselling and psychotherapy with regards to exploring the exact nature of the therapeutic relationship and much of that work might be appropriately reflected upon by professional reflexologists. Interestingly much of the research has demonstrated that the most important factor contributing to a successful therapeutic encounter is in fact the nature of the therapeutic relationship between the therapist and the client, and not the model of counselling or psychotherapy utilised.

The concept of the therapeutic relationship is probably most valued by counsellors trained in the humanistic model of *Person-Centred Theory (1951).* This particular model of counselling is defined by a rationale stating clients are the best judge of their own feelings and therefore can be the only true experts in their life. The role of the person-centred counsellor therefore is entirely supportive in essence, and the quality of the therapeutic relationship formed with the client of paramount importance. In fact in person-centred counselling the relationship is believed to have the potential to be transformative for clients in its own right.

The nature of the therapeutic relationship and how it might be playing out within a reflexology context is certainly worth some lengthy consideration. The potential quality of the relationship formed between a professional reflexologist and her client can perhaps be likened to no other occurring in the field of complementary therapies. The modality, practiced face to face and involving the powerful medium of touch might be viewed as a deeply intimate complementary practice, and as such the powerful relational dimension involved in an exchange between an attentive reflexologist and her client should not be underestimated. The proficient relational reflexologist has at her disposal not only an effective therapeutic touch and pressure modality, but also the potential of an effective therapeutic relationship, able to safely support emotional disclosure and promote self-directed change in clients.

"The way in which the reflexologist works, offering body reflections in conjunction with reflexology techniques, and the way the counsellor works using contact reflections, constitutes an allocation of the client's attention - primarily to their physical responses to their environment and to treatment, and subsequently to areas of emotional response"(Uphoff, 1999).

Within the context of a reflexology session why might the concept of a therapeutic relationship be important, and why should practitioners be striving to develop a more detailed understanding and awareness of such concepts? A third year medical student shadowing the writer in her private practice recently later reflected on his observations of the day stating, *'I'm envious of the quality of time you're able to spend with your clients'*. It is worth reflecting on what specifically this *quality of time* represents? One would hope it is perhaps representative of the warmth and depth of relationship the student witnessed between practitioner and client. Perhaps it was meant to reflect the openness and genuineness of the communications exchanged, or perhaps it was the educational and collaborative nature of the exchange itself. Ideally, this reflexology practitioner hopes her student companion was aware of each of the above.

As professional reflexologists we are extremely fortunate to be in a position to provide both the time and space required to form effective therapeutic relationships with our clients. The transformative power held in that relationship has the potential to exist far beyond the boundaries of an hour long session of reflexology and relaxation. In today's busy, time limited world, certainly from the anxious client's perspective, the beneficial effects of being held in a safe and professional relationship, whilst being touched, supported, educated and encouraged should not be underestimated.

The therapeutic relationship can provide clients with an appropriate safe and supportive space in which to freely express emotion should they wish to. It is important to remember, particularly with the sub-fertility group, that thoughts, fears and perceptions have the ability to affect the correct functioning of adrenal responses via the hypothalamus in the brain.

The fight or flight response in human beings is associated with real and perceived fear and related scientific evidence clearly dictates physical and emotional states in the body are entirely interactive in their responses. The rationale for practice in sub-fertility is strongly linked to the concept of promoting the *hospitable womb* therefore the safe nurturing of a client's emotional state should be of paramount importance to any practitioner engaging in this field.

What makes a client group vulnerable?

The phone rings and a potential new client wishes to enquire if you might be able to help him with some night cramps he has been experiencing? He thought having his feet worked on would help his circulation?

The phone rings and a potential new client wishes to enquire if you might be able to help her with Irritable Bowel Syndrome? The GP suggested she should do things to help her relax?

A phone rings and a potential new client wishes to enquire if she can book in for reflexology to help her through her upcoming IVF. She read on the internet that it has helped others and thought the relaxation might help?

On the surface it might appear from the examples given only the IVF client might require consideration if we are to be concerned about the possibility of emotional vulnerability. In reality of course any one of these clients could be emotionally vulnerable. It is important practitioners try hard not make prior judgements about the nature of why a client may be making contact or about what disclosures clients may bring to the consulting room.

When a client makes contact he or she may use the medical term IBS, for example, to describe their condition or might simply express a hope that reflexology might help them to relax and support the functioning of the digestive system. It is worth considering though, perhaps not unsurprisingly, clients experiencing a physiological stress related disorder such as IBS often *also* feel emotionally stressed when they attend for reflexology and quite frequently disclose to their practitioner why that might be. Practitioners should be therefore prepared for such disclosures and try to remain open to what might be happening within the clients real experiencing.

Why might sub-fertility clients need to be heard?

> *"The growth of complementary therapies to meet demand is unequivocal. Psychological trauma is at its most concentrated; we are suffering from overload of one kind or another and we need a safe place in which we can tell our story" March Smith (2005).*

Quite simply, sometimes clients just don't have anyone else to talk with! With regards to the sub-fertility group specifically, often a woman and her partner have simply gone past the stage of feeling anything can be gained from revisiting the situation. Sometimes women become resistant to showing their real feelings at home aware of how frustrated her partner feels about not being able to do anything more to help. Often friends and relations know only how to offer well meant positive encouragement and a woman might refrain from expressing her real frustrations and distress, fearing once again she might hear the statements 'you just need to relax' or "It'll all be fine, you'll see!'.

Women experiencing sub-fertility difficulties can therefore keep the narrative of their experiences wrapped up inside their own heads, simply because they don't have anywhere else to express what they really feel. It is not uncommon for women to talk of envy regarding yet another pregnant friend, and then follow the initial statement with *"you know you're the only person I would say that to; everyone else would think I'm awful".*

It is also worth remembering by the time a client makes contact with a reflexology practitioner she may have been engaged in a clinical and medical environment for many months or even years. Undoubtedly whilst most women receive only excellent care from the medical profession as a whole, a large portion of modern medicine is governed by time-limited appointments, effective information gathering and clinical diagnosis and treatment. Clients can sometimes feel the mechanics of medicine, no matter how scientifically astonishing, offers little to salve their inner frustrations and sadness.

Research (Kessler, Soukup, & Davis, 2001) evaluating the use of complementary therapies in the treatment of anxiety and depression demonstrated that the perceived helpfulness of the therapies was similar to that of conventional treatment. The study also demonstrated that complementary and alternative therapies are used more than conventional therapies by people with *self-defined anxiety attacks* and *severe depression*. This research was thought to demonstrate that in some cases clients may opt to engage in a modality of treatment which they feel will either be more effective for their condition or in some cases holistic treatments may be *perceived* by clients as potentially offering support in a less *authoritarian* or medically related manner. The perception a client holds with regards to the perceived outcome of treatment is often referred to as the 'placebo effect'. When relating this concept against the principles of PNI, individual perception (or the placebo effect) could be defined as relating directly to the functioning of the HPA axis.

Client expectation of the practitioner clearly plays a significant role in explaining why clients disclose, and further highlights why reflexology is in essence a relational complementary therapy. A practitioner may refer to themselves as a complementary therapist, a holistic therapist or perhaps simply as a reflexologist. Most clients however perceive our profession to be a profession of *helpers* and as such they often assume practitioners want to hear their troubles.

Indeed our profession champion's reflexology as an effective stress reliever and reflexology practitioners actively enquire about client stress levels during the consultation period. Understandably then clients can *assume* their reflexologist is interested. In essence the very signals we send out as a profession encourage our clients to disclose.

Professional and personal development

Developing a deeper understanding and appreciation of the nature of the professional therapeutic relationship can clearly help to promote a more focused awareness of the professional and ethical requirements made of practitioners wishing to engage in this sensitive field. Practitioners become better aware of how to set and maintain effective professional boundaries. A working knowledge of the therapeutic relationship can help the reflexology practitioner recognise when client disclosures are too complicated to be held safely in the consulting room and when a referral is absolutely necessary.

Understanding more about what might be happening within the therapeutic relationship can also help reflexologists develop into more confident, assured and effective professional practitioners. The reflexology practitioner who develops for example, the ability to hold a conscious thread of conversation and remain fully present in her clients experiencing, is a practitioner who is developing her empathy. This more self-aware reflexologist is also clearer about his or her motivations as a practitioner, and are more connected to how they really feel internally from day to day. This practitioner is aware of how their own personal feelings could impact on the client's experience, and therefore verbal and non-verbal responses are more considered, conscious and thought out.

This reflexologist is more present and aware in every way possible within the confines of his or her consulting room. This practitioner is developing into an effective listener and is able to provide for clients the appropriate environment required for a safe therapeutic exchange.

The building blocks of an effective therapeutic relationship

Client-centred treatment focuses on listening to clients and involving them at a profound level in their own healing and that requires good communications skills, as well as a technical proficiency in the healing modality practiced. What then does the proficient reflexologist require in addition to good technical ability and sound clinical knowledge, to be sure of providing a safe space for her clients in which positive change might occur? It would be fair to say that psychotherapists and counsellors generally agree that there are certain conditions which need to be in place for an effective therapeutic relationship to be formed. Carl Rogers, the founder of Person Centred Therapy *(1951)* referred to these as the *core conditions.*

Rogers believed *unconditional positive regard, congruence and empathy* were the foundations and qualities required of a practitioner wishing to form effective therapeutic relationships. The core therapeutic conditions required are often referred to by counsellors as *'ways of being'*.

Ideally the practitioner is striving to provide a genuine free space in which her client experiences unconditional warmth and acceptance. No demands or expectations are placed upon the client and she is free to be herself and valued as such. The practitioner hopes to demonstrate her empathic understanding of the client's unique frame of reference, mindful that for every individual the experience of life (and sub-fertility) is entirely unique, regardless the commonality of experience. The feelings of unconditionally acceptance emanating from within this supportive relationship can provide clients with the ability to begin to non-judgementally access their true thoughts and feelings and reflect more authentically upon their lives. The three core conditions necessary to provide a supportive therapeutic relationship are:

Unconditional Positive Regard: ***The client feels valued and accepted as they are: the practitioner may not approve of some of the client's actions, but the practitioner does approve of the client.***

What does it mean to unconditionally regard a person? It is a big ask really, a huge commitment surely? To find unconditional acceptance for every client we meet isn't easy admittedly. Ideally UPR develops as a part of a practitioner's life philosophy or value system. Perhaps it is best summed up as *'an acceptance of the commonality of human beings'*. Some might say we are all the same souls underneath! Of course it is sometimes difficult not to feel irritated by the talkative client who insists on telling you every detail of her life or the overly curious anxious to be your new best friend or perhaps it is the client who tends to cancel appointment regularly. Sometimes it is easy to feel disapproving or judgemental regarding the personal value set of a client, or to feel frustrated when a client neglects to make your suggested changes, or continues to engage in unhelpful behaviours. Developing unconditional positive regards encourages us to be more mindful of our own personal inner narratives and allows us to become more aware of the judgements we are holding (and we all hold some).

Attempting to be more non-judgemental can help to prevent blocks from forming in the relationship and every encounter. It can be easy to disagree with the life choices of an individual, however it is vitally important to remember that because we have not walked in that persons shoes, or experienced their particular life, we really can have no idea why a person might choose to live or behave as they do. It would be simply arrogant to believe we might know better.

Through fostering and nourishing the concept of UPR we are better able to demonstrate to our clients they are valuable and accepted, just as they are. Within the confines of the therapeutic relationship the client retains the practitioner's undivided attention, respect and focus and regards her client as absolutely important and valuable. Often when clients can experience this form of authentic acceptance from another person it can prompt an inner recognition towards developing better self care strategies, and many clients are more naturally drawn towards recognising and placing more importance upon their own value and worth.

It is worth remembering that an inner narrative belonging to the therapist, particularly of the disapproving sort, doesn't have to be voiced to become clear and apparent to a client. Facial expressions and body language can often *give our thoughts away,* so it is just not enough to remain quiet. Practitioners genuinely need to find warmth and acceptance for all of their clients so ideally a more natural feeling of general acceptance starts to become stronger than any internal disapproving voice.

No matter how good a person we might think we are, or how charitable we might feel our inner essence might be, every person is judgemental to some degree. Recognising our judgments and connecting to the innate worth and value of each individual is to develop unconditional positive regard.

Congruence: ***genuineness, authentic, being 'real' in the relationship***

This is often the most difficult core condition to define. What does it mean to be *real?* To be congruent within a therapeutic relationship might be defined as being fully present and aware in the moment; aware of our motivations, thoughts and feelings. Practitioners are striving to be real in the relationship so clients can also be real. Developing congruence can help our personal and professional development as we become more aware of the judgements we might hold when dealing with clients. In turn we are reminded to be more mindful in our interactions and reflections with clients, and so congruence can be equally helpful in developing UPR and vice versa.

As practitioners we often adopt a certain side of our personalities in a consulting room. Ideally we behave in a professional manner and our boundaries are often constructed to support this. When we are more congruent with our clients though, we can still retain a professional attitude, but we are somehow more *real* in the manner in which we relate to them. Practitioners neither attempt to wear a mask of authority nor do they want to try and be a client's best friend. The realness is demonstrated through the genuineness of the exchange and the value placed in the clients experiencing.

In order to remain within a client's frame of reference practitioners must also try to be more aware of their own thoughts and feelings. In essence, being congruent as a practitioner means thoughts, feelings and actions tie up, so that not only the client senses the realness, but the practitioner also experiences herself as fully present, real and genuine.

Congruence is often mistaken for a form of verbal honesty. Being real in the relationship doesn't mean expressing every thought that comes into your head; rather it's about being aware of thoughts and judgements, but not allowing them to prevent your presence in the relationship. To be congruent we must be real, and to be real we must be fully present and focused on the client.

Empathy: ***the ability to stand in another's frame of reference without losing sight of your own: the ability to understand what a client might be feeling. Empathy is not the same as sympathy.***

Developing Empathy: Jenny - The IVF Client

Jenny is 36 years old; employed full-time as a primary school teacher and has been trying to conceive for over two years. Jenny recently discovered she has scarring on both her fallopian tubes due to a historic pelvic infection and her consultant has explained natural conception is unlikely. Jenny was shocked by the news, and also relieved to have an explanation for her difficulties conceiving. Jenny is otherwise in good health physically, and leads a relatively normal and healthy lifestyle in relation to diet and exercise.

Jenny feels grateful to be referred directly for IVF feeling very aware time is ticking on. Feeling a little regretful about waiting until thirty six to start trying for a family, Jenny is relieved to find her local NHS authority will allow her three free attempts at IVF and she is anxious to get started as quickly as possible. Approximately two months later, two top grade embryos are returned into Jenny's perfectly lined uterus, after a textbook IVF protocol. Jenny takes the required daily progesterone medication and waits. The attempt fails and Jenny is left devastated. Jenny reads that reflexology might help and calls you looking for support.

Empathy not sympathy

The impact of reading Jenny's words will be unique for each of us. Thoughts and feelings may range from feeling very little to perhaps an appreciation of Jenny's obviously difficult situation. Some people might feel quite sad for Jenny and want to reach out and offer comfort, and for others there might simply be feelings of relief the events aren't happening to them.

Hearing other people's stories and life challenges undoubtedly impacts on each of us differently, and often our initial thoughts and feelings can be centrered around what *we* might be feeling personally. Empathy however isn't about what we feel, nor is it about offering comforting words of sympathy. Empathy is about trying to metaphorically place one's self into another person's shoes and to walk alongside them in their world, attempting to understand how it might feel for them. Empathy and empathic responses therefore are associated with *appreciating another person's frame of reference.*

What then might be an appropriate empathic conclusion to arrive at when we consider Jenny's story? If the story represents Jenny's experience then the words clearly describe her feelings of shock, anxiousness and her devastation at the failure of her IVF cycle. In practice clients also give us the clues we require to offer appropriate empathic responses, not only through their stories and words, but also their body language and facial expressions. There is a real difference though between hearing a person and listening. In normal everyday conversations (passive listening) we are often formulating our reply even as the other person is speaking. When we actively listen we give our full attention to our companion and this allows us to relate more empathically. Rogers *(1951)* described empathy as being able to walk around in another's frame of reference without losing sense of your own self. Sue Fox *(2008)* describes this relating challenge equally well:

> *"It's like listening to two stories at the same time; the one that the client is telling and the one that you are telling yourself. We listen to the words, the emotion behind them, body language, facial expression and we listen to our own body's messages; our own feelings. We learn to listen 'as if' we are the other person while at the same time listening in to our self."*

A more natural ability in demonstrating the core conditions often flourishes in line with the depth of self development and awareness a practitioner holds. The core conditions might essentially be perceived as human skills, finely tuned and intensified during focused therapeutic exchanges. Practitioner use of self within the relationship can be likened to the sum total of the core conditions, blended and demonstrated to the client through the personality and uniqueness of the practitioner. There is no mask of authority to be worn in the consulting room. Rather there exists a genuine human presentation of clarity of thought and focus, fully engaged in the world of another. Simply one human being genuinely and non-judgmentally meeting another in their world, and offering a caring, supportive ear.

Relational depth in reflexology

> *"There is nothing I can do to force this experience, but when I can relax and be close to that transcendental core of me then I may behave in strange and impulsive ways in the relationship, ways which I cannot justify rationally, which have nothing to do with my thought processes. But these strange behaviours turn out to be right in some odd way. At those moments it seems that my inner spirit has reached out and touched the inner spirit of the other."(Rogers, 1986)*

"Once in a while something extraordinary happens in the consulting room. It has nothing to do with the quality of the hands-on healing, or any obvious aspect about an average, everyday kind of appointment. It is simply an in rush of energy, a moment of connectedness which, in its hugeness has a powerful effect upon both people in the room." (March-Smith, 2005)

These two descriptions, one from a counsellor and the other from a therapist describing her body work, certainly seem to hint towards some element of commonality or overlap existing within the respective modalities. Each practitioner seems to be describing their own perception of some connection or moment occurring in the therapy room. It is this *connection* Carl Rogers might describe as a moment of *relational depth.* Rogers believed that the quality of the therapeutic relationship formed between therapist and client to be of paramount importance if there was to be any chance of working with clients at true relational depth.

As a student counsellor I recall reading for the first time about the concept of relational depth and being struck by a feeling of already understanding and that being described in the words before me. I knew instinctively on a very deep level that this theoretical counselling concept was indeed very familiar to me, and that I'd experienced such moments many times in my work as a complementary therapist. I doubt I would have been able to articulate the experience before I trained as a counsellor and I certainly wasn't aware of its relevance within my complementary work back then. Today though I believe on a profound level the theoretical concept of relational depth is very closely associated with a quality of contact often experienced between an attentive reflexologist and her client. Person-centred academics have more recently defined the concept of relational depth as:

"A feeling of profound contact and engagement with a client, in which one simultaneously experiences high and constant levels of empathy and acceptance towards that other, and relates to them in a highly transparent way. In this relationship, the client is experienced as

acknowledging one's empathy, acceptance and congruence – either implicitly or explicitly – and is experienced as fully congruent in that moment." (Mearns & Thorne (2007)

Brian Thorne, another well know person-centred academic, known to counsellors for his passionate writing involving the spiritual nature of some therapeutic encounters, believes moments of relational depth can be achieved simply as a result of an encounter between two human beings. In his book *The Mystical Power of Person-Centred Counselling* (2002) Thorne states:

"All that is required is a preparedness for two people to meet at relational depth and for one to be thoroughly schooled in the practice of offering the core conditions to herself and to the other who seeks her help."

Taken out of context Thorne's statement might allow us to believe moments of relational depth happen every time two human beings come into contact. Whilst moments of relational depth between people do indeed happen in everyday life, it still remains a relatively rare occurrence for any individual to experience such a singular focus of attention concerned with her life and experiencing. The confines of any therapeutic session where focus is placed on the client's needs, and through which a therapeutic relationship can be formed can, under favourable circumstances, produce transformative moments of relational depth.

What does relational depth achieve?

"The experience of relational depth opens up channels for understanding and profound connectedness which can transform a person's sense of self and engender new hope and meaning." (Thorne, 2002)

Ideally experiencing relational depth from a client's perspective relates to being really seen and heard. Clients feel understood, acknowledged, cherished and some even say prized. Sometimes a client can feel as though a moment in time stands still and everything suddenly becomes a little clearer. In essence, these moments of relational depth happen when a person who wants to be helped is on the receiving end of unconditional, positive regard, empathy and congruence. Given the freedom to express their hopes, fears and frustrations, clients can often come to find moments of deep love and new appreciation for their own situation. Positive changes are often born from this new place of acceptance and self love.

Sub-fertility clients in particular can find through a supportive relationship, a renewed sense of dedication towards their own personal needs. In turn these more pro-active feelings can induce increased feelings of being in more in control, thus helping to reduce feelings of stress and anxiety, potentially calming autonomic stress responses in the body.

Engaging with clients on more than a superficial level and trying to look past what Brian Thorne *(2002)* refers to as a *manualised set of instructions,* requires a brave practitioner indeed. It takes a strong heart to offer clients a place to freely sob and not be overcome with a desire to offer hugs and comfort in return. It's not always easy to remain composed when a client talks about not wanting her young step son in her home during her upcoming IVF, or you find you are listening to a client talk in a negative manner about her tired pregnant friend.

Social norms and assumed appropriate behaviour have a tendency to block more authentic relationships. Clients often maintain a professional image and present only a part of their persona to work colleagues and employers. A slightly different face might be applied when doing the weekly shop or collecting the dry cleaning. Clients may show a little more of themselves to close family or friends, but rarely do clients show or even connect with their whole self. Within the context of a focused relational reflexology encounter clients are given that space to be wholly themselves. They may express whatever they want to, in any manner the wish to and anything they do express is held in high value.

The focus of any relational encounter from the practitioner's perspective leans towards promoting the collective, dynamic core conditions. The client who chooses to react to these core conditions, and able to perceive the realness of the practitioner, can often in turn relate to her own experiences in a more authentic and caring manner. Whilst the focus for the practitioner might be towards providing the core conditions, one should not be under the illusion clients are focused upon the same goal. The clients focus and attention should be rightly steered towards what they might be experiencing both generally, and within the session itself.

Understanding why human beings are so fond of reflexologists and ready to disclose to practitioners their deep fears and wishes for the future clearly requires and deserves more attention. Perhaps because many reflexologists offer natural relating skills and a genuine interest in the clients experiences, combined with the equally beneficially elements of a deeply relaxing pressure therapy and intimate therapeutic touch, the modality offers a powerful recipe for producing the perfect environment for wonderfully therapeutic moments of relational depth.

Ideally in the future more will be written regarding the concept of the relationship and relational depth within reflexology and undoubtedly long words and fancy paragraphs used to define such concepts. Regardless of the complexity of any information we might need to digest it can often prove wise to begin constructing our understanding using the most simplified definition available. If I were being asked to define the concept of relational depth within my reflexology practice, and explain why it happens, I would reply simply: *"I am present; I care and my clients can feel it."*

Client leads, practitioner follows

How do we keep the brakes working efficiently within this new relating relationship? How do we ensure reflexology practitioners don't step too far outside their professional boundaries? After all, reflexologists are not professional counsellors. Earlier in the chapter we referred to the person-centred concept which states the client is the only true expert in their life and experiencing. As we have also explored it is perhaps wise to adopt the same stance as budding relational reflexologists, and strive to relate with our clients in an entirely empathetic manner. Empathy ensuring above all we remain focused within our client's unique frame of reference at all times.

The client *must* retain autonomy in the relationship and direct the content of the session according to her own needs. The use of clarifying and open questioning can indeed be appropriate during active listening, often helping to draw out a more complete picture to support a practitioners empathetic understanding, in essence however the practitioners role is to listen, empathise and offer supportive reflective responses and support.

This doesn't mean though as practitioners we can't be human! It is absolutely fine to enquire directly, for example, how a client is managing and coping during her IVF cycle. The practitioner who is prepared for a possible emotional response to such a question and ready to manage an appropriately reflective and empathic response would be viewed as a practitioner respecting the client's whole experience. This practitioner is simply giving voice to his or her concern and awareness, and relating to the clients experience authentically. This practitioner is responding as a human being and demonstrating care for the client within the boundaries of a safe therapeutic relationship.

There seems to exist within the reflexology industry an odd attitude that emotional content is somehow inappropriate and should be wholly avoided where possible. Emotional content is in reality an integral element of the human experience and therefore for most people a shared experience. Dealing with emotional content or indeed promoting an environment in which emotions might be disclosed should not be viewed in the same light as metaphorically opening a can of worms.

Relational reflexology is primarily concerned with offering support and a safe therapeutic environment to women with sub-fertility issues, as well as other emotionally vulnerable groups. Of course practitioners must develop an understanding of when a referral to a professional counsellor might be necessary, but it would be wrong to imagine emotions should only be expressed in a counselling room. To do so would be to deny the reality of the human experience, and to dismiss entirely the innate ability of one human being to appreciate emotional distress in another and react appropriately. Sub-fertility reflexology clients rarely require formal structured counselling. They require instead care support, education and encouragement.

Ideally the relationship and any exchange between a reflexologist and her client should be of a supportive and collaborative nature. Within this relationship greater reliance can be placed on existential responsibility and self-directed change stemming from the client. In order for clients to make necessary lifestyle changes they often have to be given detailed information and this information is far more likely to be heard, digested and acted upon if delivered within a space of acceptance, collaboration and care.

Practitioners must be mindful of remaining empathetic to a client's unique frame of reference at all times. It does not matter what a practitioner might think, feel or do personally in any given situation. Power and authority have no place in the therapeutic relationship. The role of the relational reflexologist is entirely supportive and practitioners must respect the existential choice and autonomy of the client.

Developing reflective and active listening skills

What does it mean then to be an empathic skilled listener? Active listening skills are required in many professions and as part of many human interactions. When we really *hear* a person and give them our full attention, trying hard to understand what life might be like from their point of view, we honour that individual's experience, and place real importance upon it. Experiencing this quality of non-judgemental attention from a skilled listener, being aware of no pressure to be anything other than present in the moment, can often feel quite transformative for clients.

Of course counselling as a therapeutic intervention and the use of counselling skills are not the same thing. The advanced skills and theoretical knowledge possessed by trained counsellors pertaining to emotional human development and behaviours means counselling is a highly skilled intervention, and one which should only to be practiced by those qualified to do so. However, the use of active and reflective listening skills might be viewed as highly appropriate and entirely valuable within the context of a reflexology session, and particularly so with the anxious sub-fertility client.

Non-verbal communication

NVC (non verbal communication), such as body language and eye contact are important skills to become aware of in an active listening encounter. Practitioners should strive not only to become more aware of what their own body language might be expressing, but also more aware of the whole client during treatment. Practitioners should try to be aware of physical reactions, facial expressions and posture.

Consider for a moment the fidgeting client, her hands moving from her lap to the sides of the chair, or perhaps the client who twiddles her thumbs nervously. A different client may lie perfectly still and silently throughout the reflexology treatment but the practitioner becomes aware the client has started to cry. Reflecting such observations gently to clients can be viewed as acknowledging attentively a real connection to the clients experiencing. The use of reflecting what a practitioner can see, or might perceive in a clients body language or indeed in response to a verbal disclosure, provides the practitioner with a reflective intervention which can be experienced as *affirming* of the clients experience, and often reflections such as these can help clients to focus more even more directly and authentically on their own felt sense and real experiencing.

Reflection and paraphrasing as an empathic tool

The use of reflection as a verbal tool can be a useful and appropriate skill. A verbal reflection is neither a question nor a statement of fact, but more a simple reflection of what the listener can see, hear or feel. If the practitioner's observation is incorrect then clients will often say so, quickly often moving on to clarify what they *are* feeling. Sometimes therefore even incorrect reflective responses can help a client focus more authentically on what they are feeling. For example, perhaps the practitioner comments on how her client's facial expression has changed and that she now looks quite sad.

Practitioner: *"It feels like all of a sudden you've become quite sad. Your facial expression has changed".*

Client: *I think I just realised as I relaxed here how tired I really feel.*

Practitioner: *"You've had a lot to deal with lately"*

Client: *"Yes, I just hate all this IVF stuff. I just wanted to have a baby".*

Practitioner: *"It sounds like you're quite fed up by the whole thing".*

Client: "*It takes over everything. My head, my thoughts and my time"*

Practitioner: *The experience has taken its toll on you emotionally?"*

Client: *Yes, it certainly has. It's been really difficult". *Client starts to sob quietly**

The example given here asks neither a question nor does it make a definite statement, instead it is simply a reflection of what the listener can see or might hear or feel. A different client may perhaps openly and verbally express her frustration as she walks through the consulting room door and again for the practitioner to pause and communicate her understanding can be equally affirming for the client.

Practitioner: *"It sounds as though you've been through a lot this week? The feelings of frustration are building up and spilling out into everyday life?*

Client: *"Yes, I've been so bad tempered and snappy. My poor husband has had it in the neck all week, and I think my boss hates me."*

Practitioner: *It sounds like it's becoming more difficult for you to separate your longing for a baby from everyday life?*

Client: *"It is. Every day it seems to get harder" *Sighs**

Sometimes active listening and empathy are related to exploring the meaning behind a statement. Perhaps a practitioner is aware of feeling anxious herself as she listens to her client relate her story. The client may never actually use the word anxious in her description, but the practitioner might reflect what she is aware of feeling, for example:

Practitioner: *"As I listen to you talk of your experience I've become aware of feeling quite anxious; in fact my tummy feels as though its turning cartwheels right now. I wonder if that's how this whole experience feels for you."*

This example of a reflective response is neither guess work, nor is it merely an account of how the practitioner thinks she might feel in the same situation. This response is ideally born from a practitioner consciously becoming more aware of what she is feeling in her own body, accessing her own felt sense as she listens to her client.

These types of empathic reflections can be quite difficult to judge initially and it is not unusual to feel worried the reflection might be entirely incorrect. The good news is where empathy is concerned, the most important element is a willingness to understand and appreciate another's experience. Practitioners should learn to trust in the person they are relating with to know deep inside how they *really* feel. What matters to the client is they know the practitioner is trying hard to understand.

Similarly, paraphrasing can be useful in an active listening context. Paraphrasing can also be used to help the listener clarify or double check an interpretation and demonstrate empathic understanding of what a client may have expressed using different words:

Client: *"I'm so angry! If it isn't bad enough I have to deal with not getting pregnant my referral letter has gone missing, and now I'll have to wait another two months for an appointment. I don't have time to waste. Why is this happening to me?"*

Practitioner: *"It sounds like you're feeling really frustrated by having to wait even longer to see the consultant?"*

Client: *"I am frustrated. The whole thing frustrates me. I feel so wound up all the time."*

Practitioner: *"Well I think maybe that's understandable. It sounds like you've been through a lot."*

Client: "I have." *Sighs*

Open and clarifying questions

The use of both open and clarifying questions can be immensely useful to practitioners as they allow us to deepen our understanding and also double check meaning. Open questions allow for more than a simple *yes or no* reply and can give clients more space to form a more accurate, detailed reply. Most complementary therapist are rather adept at utilising open questions, as we often learn quickly during consultation periods that closed questions don't always bring forth the information required. Open and clarifying questions often therefore start with words like when, where, how and why.

Blocks to the relationship

The unwilling client

There are undoubtedly sub-fertility clients who only wish to engage in reflexology to experience a session of focused quiet and relaxation. Practitioners should NEVER attempt to force such clients into conversation or expect emotional disclosure. If a client chooses to remain silent, or indeed fall into quiet reflective periods during a session, the practitioner must respect the client's autonomy to do so.

External influences

A room too cold, warm, noisy or even overly cluttered can present difficulties. Most complementary therapists are well versed in how to provide an appropriate physical environment, however with this particular client group there are additional factors worth consideration. Home visits are generally not advised. Many practitioners are already aware of the difficulties existing relating to control of environment when visiting clients at home. Practitioners are less able to stop the phone ringing or prevent other disruptions during sessions. Additionally clients can often find it more difficult to relax when reminded of the huge pile of ironing on the dining room table or the dog is barking to be let out. Practitioners who are more able to provide a more controlled, peaceful and undisturbed physical environment for their clients are far more likely to be able to promote an appropriate environment more conducive to producing authentic relational exchanges.

Practitioner physical and emotional health

Poor health, pain and general illness in practitioners can also hinder the development of therapeutic relationships, as can deep emotional burdens.

Practitioners who find themselves physically in poor health are best advised to postpone sessions with vulnerable clients until such a time as good health returns. Concerning the emotional health of a practitioner specifically, we might consider this in two parts. Firstly there are those more short term emotional strains such as bereavement, divorce and relationship problems, or any other difficulty which can prevent practitioners from focusing on clients needs effectively and which can hinder the development of the therapeutic relationship. Until such a time as the practitioner can be sure of feeling personally more emotionally balanced and therefore able to be more fully present within in the relationship, sessions should be discontinued and clients ideally referred to an appropriate alternative practitioner. This allows the practitioner space and time to focus on self care and ensures the emotional safety of the client.

The wounded healer

The second element to consider relates to the general emotional disposition of the practitioner. There is an interesting phenomenon occurs in professions where empathy is required and encouraged. Perhaps the best way to consider this phenomenon would be to enquire why you, the reader, trained as a reflexologist? The theme in essence relates to the concept of a 'wounded healer'. Studies have demonstrated that in many cases individuals who have chosen to follow careers paths involving caring or helping as an element have, *"often as children experienced loneliness, illness, bereavement or the need to look after others"* March-Smith (2005). Researchers have suggested that with such children the ability to empathise has often developed to such a degree in childhood that as adults these individuals somehow feel compelled to care for others in some capacity and are often drawn towards more therapeutic professions.

"the presence of such a 'wound' in a healer gives them an excellent basis from which to understand and empathise with the wounds of clients." McLoud (1998)

Whilst certainly no assumption can be made that all reflexologists possess such an inner *wound,* the concept does demonstrate a requirement for good levels of self awareness in professional reflexology practitioners. Practitioners more aware of their inner motivations and drives are potentially in less danger of exhausting their own personal energy and more able to maintain appropriate professional boundaries and offer appropriate reflective responses.

Practitioner attitudes and inner narrative

False empathy might be defined as believing your reactions or feelings might be exactly the same as your clients and is therefore associated with assumption and not with listening empathically. Believing for example a client should cry more, or to perhaps to assume more wealthy people don't feel quite so deeply would be to think in a judgemental manner. Practitioners should always strive to relate to clients empathically, promoting a more non-judgmental and accurate assessment of a clients unique frame of reference.

Some theorists have attempted to provide a scale for the concept of empathy and it can be useful to consider this information as we develop our skills in delivering appropriate empathic responses:

Client: **Quietly sobbing after disclosing her feelings of pain regarding the loss of a much wanted pregnancy**

Practitioner: *"I understand how it feels to lose something you loved. My dog died recently and he was a very special part of my life. I'll miss him forever."*

A response of this nature clearly demonstrates a lack of any deep meaningful empathy or understanding. Whilst the practitioners grief may be very real and the experience deeply painful, within a therapeutic context, as an empathic response it is neither relevant nor appropriate. A response of this nature, whilst admittedly on a very basic level could be considered as loosely empathic (grief theme), does not suggest empathy of a deep enough level (from within the client's frame of reference) to achieve moments of any real relational depth. A more appropriate response for example, might be:

Practitioner: *"I can sense from your words and tears how deeply this loss has affected you. Your sadness seems very present, even now in this room."*

The two responses demonstrate empathy must be of a depth appropriately reflective of appreciating the client's unique frame of reference.

Endings

Endings are related to professional boundaries. Endings are generally easier to deal with if they have been acknowledged during the initial verbal contracting between a practitioner and a client. Practitioners should strive to agree on the focus and duration of sessions by the end of the consultation period, ensuring this verbal contract is reassessed regularly to ensure session focus remains with the client's needs. This is particularly important when dealing with natural sub-fertility clients who can often require a longer term session plan, and require regular re-assessment of progress relating to physiological and experiential change.

The concept of endings within complementary and holistic fields is worth consideration. Many clients continue to visit their complementary practitioners monthly, sometimes long after an initial six to eight week intensive period of treatment has ended. The sub-fertility client group however does not fall into this category generally. Endings happily come about in many cases because a client achieves pregnancy and in these situations practitioners can often experience intense feelings of happiness and genuine satisfaction. However, the work can also present practitioners with another set of more complex and challenging emotions.

Sometimes practitioners are left experiencing real feelings of sadness and frustration when clients don't reach their goal. Feelings of sadness can arise when a practitioner who misses the once regular slot with the client she felt so fond of, and sometimes it is the client who misses the practitioner. It is not uncommon for example, for clients to feel they have lost a trusted friend at the end of intervention.

Any practitioner who chooses to engage in sub-fertility work must respect the deep bond of trust which can be formed between a practitioner and sub-fertility client. The relationship, no matter how short lived can be both intense and intimate, and practitioners can undoubtedly experience a deep sense of privilege being involved in something so life changing for clients. Practitioners must learn also however, with such intensity and privileged access into the emotional realm of another lies the challenge of *letting go*, and that means sometimes never hearing from a client again. The requirement therefore for clear boundaries in practice and appropriate practitioner self development once again comes into focus.

Practitioner self awareness

Clearly practitioner self awareness is of paramount importance if the therapeutic core conditions are to be given space to flourish. The concept of unconditional positive regard requires practitioners to develop a better awareness of their personal judgements and opinions whilst encouraging the development of genuine kinship with our fellow human beings. Congruence requires the practitioner to be more confident in her own skin, and able to trust her instincts and motivations, whilst empathy demands we recognise the difference between our feelings and reactions and the feeling and reactions of our clients. Good counsellors work on their own self development as much as they do in developing a sound theoretical understanding of their therapeutic modality and it would seem appropriate reflexology practitioners wishing to engage with any vulnerable client group should do the same. Completing a counselling skills course or engaging with a supportive local counseling supervisor can provide practitioners with a space for personal exploration, emotional support and help to develop increased practitioner self awareness.

Professional supervision

Holding safely the emotional strains of another human being can be challenging on both an ethical and a personal front. Practitioner's who choose to engage with a local experienced counsellor in a supervisory capacity, are promoting professional standards within their own practice, and helping to ensure both client and practitioner remain safe. The concept of professional supervision is undervalued by complementary therapists in general. Experiencing good supervision can install confidence in a practitioner.

> *"A good supervisor is a resource, a shoulder to cry on, a listening ear, and provides time to be still and listen to your inner voice."(Fox, 2008)*

Whilst peer supervision can indeed also be useful and allow practitioners to learn from one another and share experiences, the additional benefits derived from engaging with a professionally qualified supervisor can be enormous. Practitioners might consider coming together and engaging in a group supervision session, with the financial cost of engaging with the supervisor shared amongst the group. Professional supervisors are trained in focusing attention on the practitioner(s) and within this relationship the work of the practitioner and any feeling around the work are of primary concern. Supervision can be helpful in re-defining the boundaries of a therapeutic relationship, ensuring relationships remain professional. It can also help with issues emerging from dealing with the weight of client's emotional content or issues which arise in the practitioner because of transference or counter-transference.

Transference and counter-transference

Transference literally means to *"carry across."* (Fox, 2008). Transference and counter-transference can be defined as the unconscious transference of feelings or attitudes of a person from the past, onto a person in the present, and the concept is widely accepted as an element existing within many therapeutic relationships. Unconscious transference in the relationship might display, for example, in a client who transfers feelings about authority or perhaps a mother figure onto the practitioner. The practitioner's responsibility is to remain aware and alert to such possibilities. Practitioners can equally sometimes develop feelings of responsibility for their clients and this can also potentially hinder the development of client autonomy and the possibility of self directed change.

Transference can occur simply because the behaviours or even the look of an individual can remind us of past relationships. Transference happens entirely unconsciously and for those practitioners who wish to work with more vulnerable client groups developing an understanding of such and its potential influence within therapeutic encounters is highly recommended. Supervision can expertly support practitioners working through such issues, ensuring professional relationships and therapeutic encounters remain focused in the client's best interests. A well qualified and experienced professional supervisor can certainly help practitioners develop a more rounded appreciation of such issues.

Sourcing structured professional supervision

Another weighty challenge facing the future of professional reflexology is that of how to encourage and introduce the concept of structured professional supervision. Given the obvious complexity of the reflexology package professional practitioners engaging with vulnerable clients groups should ideally be sourcing professional support from within the field of counselling and psychotherapy. Unfortunately however, the concept of *touch* remains a rather thorny issue for talking therapists.

Generally touch is not promoted within counselling and psychotherapy settings, with some research demonstrating a real fear amongst talking therapists regarding their use of touch within a therapeutic context. The attitude seems to be connected to a concern that touch might somehow be perceived or contextualised as sexual or inappropriate; (Rutter, 1989); (Stenzel & Rupert, 2004); (Galton, 2006). Other research (Geib, 1998) highlighted a trend with therapists who had *historically* used touch with clients but *"felt unable to talk about it to anybody"*. A detailed analysis of the use of touch in counselling and psychotherapy found that the most common forms of touch to be utilised in a counselling setting remained as, *"handshakes and hugs*" and that female therapists were *"significantly more likely only to hug female clients*." (Williams, Clarke, & Gibson, 2011).

Clearly the manner in which touch is currently perceived within counselling and psychotherapy presents potential complications for relational reflexologists. Many professional counselling supervisors might presently be reluctant to engage with a practitioner utilising touch as a central component of intervention, sadly believing they could not offer anything worthwhile. Some might even perhaps be a little offended by the notion clients might choose to share their emotions outside of a counselling room. Whilst there are of course some professional supervisors with duel experience and training, who might perhaps feel more comfortable discussing touch related topics, sadly at present, they are few in number.

Until such a time as reflexology practitioners are able to provide adequate professional supervision from within the reflexology industry professional practitioners must continue to attempt find support from external sources. As an industry we must therefore strive to gain increased professional respect and support from those qualified in providing professional psychological support and supervision. This stance will undoubtedly be more easily achieved if practitioners can go on to develop a more extensive academic and clinical knowledge base capable of appreciating the multi-dimensional complexity of the reflexology package.

It is only through appropriate practitioner education that our profession can develop these important professional relationships. Through identifying common theoretical ground and developing a shared therapeutic language, the reflexology profession will be far better positioned to encourage the professional counselling and psychotherapy world to support our modality and its practitioners.

Summary

The use of active and reflective listening skills within a reflexology session can be experienced as very affirming for clients. Experiencing feelings of being valued within the therapeutic relationship can often be transformative. Therapeutic relationships of this type can help clients to re-connect more fully with their own bodies and to accept their real feelings and experiences often in turn prompting self-directed change and an increased sense of regaining control.

The effects these changes can promote in a client's physiological and emotional well-being are rarely anything other than positive. It is essential however practitioners remain aware of the ethical responsibility of signposting clients to a professional counsellor should emotional strains be too challenging to hold safely in the therapy room. The nature of this work and the client group is clearly delicate, and the ethical responsibility lies with the practitioner to ensure both he or she, in addition to the client, remain safe at all times.

Developing skills which broaden the professional skills set, and therefore the effectiveness of a practitioner within the confines of her consulting room, rarely have anything other than a positive effect, both professionally and personally. As holistic and complementary practitioner's one important element of our work dictates appropriate steps are taken regarding self care. Developing the skills involved required to build effective therapeutic relationships necessitates a deep element of practitioner self development. Better self care is often born from such newly acquired information for both clients and practitioners alike.

Unconditional positive regard, congruence and empathy are innately human skills and can perhaps be defined within a relational reflexology context as simply a natural element morphed into being during those indefinable precious moments when two individuals genuinely meet and touch within the life and experience of one. Moments of relational depth happen in reflexology sessions principally because reflexologists *care*.

The question of how to hold this relational connection safely, for both practitioners and clients alike, provides a solid rationale for actively encouraging those professional reflexologists who engage with vulnerable client groups to develop more fully their professional relating skills, and engage in deeper levels of self development and appropriate professional supervision.

CHAPTER FIVE

CLINICAL INFORMATION

Conception and early pregnancy

Fertilisation

Fertilisation can be defined as the joining of a sperm *(gamete)* and a mature egg *(ovum).* It's estimated only 100/4million sperm reach the typical fertilisation site, the fallopian tubes. To penetrate the egg the sperm must break through two barriers surrounding the ovum, the corona radiata and the zona pellucida. On reaching the plasma membrane of the egg, a reaction is initiated which prevents further sperm from breaking through to the egg membrane. Once inside the sperm sheds its tail and the two nuclei *(23 chromosomes from the sperm and 23 chromosomes from the ovum)* fuse and develop into a *zygote.* The chromosomes carry the generic information required as the building blocks of life. The sex of the baby is determined by male gametes due to female ovum carrying only X sex chromosomes, whilst sperm carries both X andY sex chromosomes.

Pre-embryonic period

The zygote begins a process of dividing by mitosis until it reaches 16 cells referred to as a *morula.* The morula begins to fills with fluid and the cells form two separate groups called a *blastocyst.* The embryoblast makes up the inner layer of cells, developing into the foetus, and the outer layer is called a *trophoblast* and this develops into part of the placenta. Once in contact with the thickened endometrium the trophoblast utilises specialised cells designed to spread and grown into the endometrium and assist with implantation.

Implantation

The blastocyst secretes hCG hormones to maintain the corpus luteum which in turn secretes progesterone, maintaining the endometrial lining of the uterus and helping to ensure the blastocyst remains embedded within the endometrium. As the placenta begins to form it takes responsibility for producing progesterone. The embryoblast within the blastocyst forms 3 primary germ layers: the *ectoderm*, *mesoderm*, and *endoderm*. The ectoderm forms the epidermis of skin, hair, nails, sweat glands, tooth enamel, lining of oral cavity, anal cavity and vagina, brain, sensory organs, lens of eye and epithelium of conjunctiva, pituitary gland and adrenal medulla. The mesoderm forms the kidneys, blood vessels, muscle tissues, connective tissue, adrenal cortex and reproductive organs. The endoderm forms the digestive tract, lungs, tonsils, liver, pancreas, thyroid, parathyroid, anterior pituitary and thymus glands and urogenital systems.

Formation of the placenta and amniotic fluid

The formation of fetal and maternal tissue makes the functional unit called the *placenta*. The placenta allows for nutrients and waste products to diffuse between the fetal blood system and that of the mother. The *amnion* is a membranous attached to the placenta which fills with water (amniotic fluid) around two weeks after fertilization and provides protection and buoyancy for the developing embryo. The amniotic fluid eventually contains vital nutrients which aid in the growth of the fetus, and in the later stages of pregnancy the amniotic fluid is utilised to prepare the digestive organs for function *(swallowing the fluid)*, and with lung development *(breathing the fluid in)*.

For most women the first sign of pregnancy is a missed period *(menses)*. This occurs because the blastocyst triggers the release of **hCG** *(human chorionic gonadotropin)*, the hormone recognised by pregnancy tests. Human pregnancy lasts approximately 40 weeks. The medical term for a developing baby is *embryo* (early weeks) and from then onwards, until birth a *fetus*.

Sub-fertility - a definition

Experts believe the chance of spontaneous conception occurring in the first month of active trying lies at around 30%. Thereafter the chance falls to around 5% by the end of the first active year. Sub-fertility is defined as failure to conceive after one year of regular sexual intercourse. A natural reduction in fertility occurs in women in their late 30s and early 40s, with the chance of conceiving for women between 35-39 years half that of women aged 19-26. Genetic defects found in older sperm and oocytes (immature ovum) are thought to impair gamete (sperm) function and embryonic development. Sub-fertility can be clinically defined as:

Primary sub-fertility*: a delay for couples with no previous pregnancies*

Secondary sub-fertility: ***a delay for a couple who have previously conceived; but the pregnancy may not have been successful (ectopic pregnancy or miscarriage).***

Research has demonstrated that the ovulatory cycle lasts approximately six days, with optimum levels peaking 2 days before ovulation and dipping by the day of ovulation. The chance of conception is therefore increased if sperm is deposited into the genital tract before ovulation. Experts also believe BMI (body mass index) impacts on sub-fertility with research demonstrating women are more likely to achieve conception with a BMI of >20 <30.

Smoking, caffeine and recreational drugs are also believed to reduce the chance of natural conception. Whilst it is difficult for researchers to ascertain the precise effects of smoking it has been estimated that smokers are 3.4 times more likely to take 12 months or more to conceive. Researchers also believe increased sub-fertility rates may be associated with factors such as a rise in environmental oestrogentic pollutants, correlating with a recent decline in sperm counts in Europe and North America.

Clinical conditions relating to sub-fertility

Sub-fertility issues can be broadly categorised as disorders relating to ovulation, tubal damage, unexplained, male factors and other hormonally related conditions such as endometriosis.

Amenorrhea

The generic term used to refer to the absence of a woman's menstrual period. Amenorrhea is not a disease, rather it is the generic name given simply to the symptom of absent menstruation. Secondary amenorrhea is more common and refers to either the temporary or permanent ending of periods in a woman who has menstruated normally in the past. Many women miss a period occasionally however amenorrhea only clinically occurs if a woman misses three or more periods in succession.

Primary amenorrhea is a rare occurrence in a therapist's private practice as it relates specifically to the failure to start to menstruate by the age of 16. It can sometimes be difficult to find the cause of amenorrhea. The GP will often perform blood tests to check for signs of androgen excess, oestrogen deficiency or other problems associated with the endocrine system such as thyroid disorders. Typical causes of secondary amenorrhea might include:

- excessive weight loss such as that which occurs as a result of anorexia nervosa or bulimia
- excessive weight gain or general poor diet
- emotional stress or depression

- stopping birth control
- strenuous physical exercise
- hypothyroidism
- PCOS (Poly Cystic Ovarian Syndrome)

Anovulation

Ovulation disorders occur in around 30% of women experiencing sub-fertility problems and often present with irregular periods (oligomenorrhoea) or an absence of periods (amenorrhea).

PCOS (Polycystic Ovarian Syndrome)

Polycystic ovary syndrome (PCOS) is a increasingly common female endocrine disorder in women of reproductive age and believed to be one of the leading causes of sub-fertility in the West. As well as menstrual difficulties women with PCOS also experience high levels of androgens (masculinising hormones) in the body. Symptoms are adult acne, hirsutism (hair growth), androgynous alopecia (hair loss), lethargy, depression and in some cases sub-fertility. There is also a strong link between PCOS and insulin resistance, further linked to a tendency in these women towards weight gain and central obesity and type II diabetes, which in turn can increase the chance of developing anovulation.

Clinical diagnosis and treatment for PCOS

Not all women with PCOS however have polycystic ovaries (PCO), nor do all women with ovarian cysts have PCOS and so the symptoms and severity of the syndrome vary greatly among affected women. A clinical diagnosis of PCOS is normally made in a woman experiencing anovulation through blood tests to confirm excessive androgen levels and check on the concentrations of luteinising hormone, follicle stimulating hormone and estradiol. Additional a svaginal ultrasound exam of the pelvis can be carried out to confirm the presence of cysts.

In the first instance women with PCOS are advised to lose weight where necessary. One front-line medical treatment utilised to treat PCOS is an insulin sensitising medication called Metformin which acts to support the pancreas (the organ which secretes the hormone insulin). Once insulin resistance in the body is corrected and rebalanced; the endocrine system in general seems to stabilise and ovulation and the menstrual cycle often spontaneously restart. Symptomatic treatments of PCOS might include the use of anti-androgens, and/or steroid hormones such as the oral contraceptive. Relating to the treatment of PCOS related sub-fertility the use of chomiphene citrate is often considered to induce ovulation: in addition to IVF depending on the age of the woman.

Tubal sub-fertility

Fallopian tubes are highly specialised organs responsible for picking up and transporting eggs, sperm and embryos. Eggs are fertilised in the fallopian and the first stages of embryo development occur in the tubes. Scar tissue present in the fallopian tubes occurring as a result of historic PID (pelvic inflammatory disease) can hinder egg pickup and transport, fertilisation and then transportation of the embryo to the uterus. Endometriosis can also leave scar tissue, as can previous pelvic surgery. Fallopian tubes can be lost entirely as a result of tubal ectopic pregnancy, which is also more common in women with scarred fallopian tubes. In many cases of tubal sub-fertility women are referred directly for IVF after a clinical diagnosis.

Dysmenorrhea

Dysmenorrhea is not a disease rather it is the generic name given to excessive menstrual pain which has a tendency to interfere with normal daily routines and activities. Dysmenorrhea can often co-exist with heavy menstrual bleeding, known as Menorrhagia. Primary dysmenorrhea is menstrual pain in otherwise healthy women normally occurring from the onset of menstruation and where no other underlying medical condition is present. Secondary dysmenorrhea is menstrual pain which develops later in women who had normal menstrual cycles and is often related with medical conditions affecting the uterus or pelvis. The GP may perform blood test of refer the patient using an exploratory laparoscopy or pelvic scan. Typical causes of secondary dysmenorrhea might include: endometriosis ovarian cysts uterine fibroids, pelvic inflammatory disease, copper IUD.

Endometriosis

Endometriosis is a medical condition in which cells from the lining of the uterus (endometrium) appear and grow outside of the uterine cavity and present in 20-40% of women who present with sub-fertility. The endometrial cells react to hormonal changes and behave in a similar manner to cells found inside the uterus. The most common areas for these cells to found are in the fallopian tubes, ovaries, bladder, bowel, vagina or rectum. Endometriosis is often a chronic condition which causes painful and/or heavy menstrual periods. The condition can also be responsible for severe pelvic, abdominal and lower back pain as well as a lack of energy, and in severe cases depression and fertility problems. Some women however suffer few or no symptoms at all and a diagnosis might only be made as a result of deeper investigation such as a laparoscopy.

The cause of endometriosis is not fully known. The most common theory is that cells from the womb lining (endometrium) do not leave the body properly during the menstrual cycle and instead embed onto the organs of the pelvis. Each month because the endometrial cells behave in the same way as those that line the uterus, they go through the same process of thickening and shedding, and his can lead to pain, swelling and even damage to the fallopian tubes or ovaries (known as endometriotic lesions).

Complications resulting from endometriosis can include internal scarring, adhesions, pelvic and ovarian cysts, bowel obstruction and pelvic adhesions. Infertility can often be related to scar tissue and anatomical distortions caused by the endometrial cells; however, it's thought endometriosis may also interfere in more subtle ways: in that endometriotic lesions may release other factors (inflammatory cytokines and other chemical agents) that somehow interfere with reproduction.

Clinical diagnosis and treatment for endometriosis

Laparoscopy: a commonly used keyhole surgery procedure used to diagnose endometriosis.

Topical Analgesia: Non-steroid anti-inflammatory drugs (NSAID), such as ibuprofen or codeine, are often used to treat the pain associated with endometriosis, principally because they act against the inflammation (swelling) caused by endometriosis, as well as helping to ease pain and discomfort.

Hormones: The aim of hormone treatments (GnRH) is to limit or stop the production of oestrogen in the body and therefore reduce any stimulating effect oestrogen has on the growth of the endometrial tissue. Hormone treatments however have no effect on endometrial lesions and do little to improve fertility.

Surgery: A laparoscopy is a commonly used keyhole surgery procedure used to diagnose and treat endometriosis and related ovarian cysts. All grades of endometriosis can be successfully treated with this minimally invasive technique. Heat, lasers or an electric current are applied to destroy the affected tissue. A laparotomy is a less common major surgery only used if the endometriosis is severe and extensive. Although both types of surgery can often relieve symptoms temporarily it's not uncommon for symptoms to recur, particularly if some endometrial cell tissue is left behind during surgery, and for this reason it's not uncommon for women suffering from severe endometriosis to undergo several laparoscopies across her fertile years.

Fibroids

Fibroids are benign tumours of the myometrium and occur in 30% of women are are estimated to have a detrimental effect of fertility in up to 10% of women. Fibroids can be reduced in size temporarily by hormonal medications, such as gonodatrophin releasing analogues (GnRH), however once re-exposed to a more oestrogen rich environment they often start to grow again. Surgical removal of larger fibroids is often carried out after a period of shrinking brought about through the administration of GnRH medication.

Unexplained/non-specific infertility

Whilst unexplained infertility is not a medically diagnosed condition in the traditional sense but it does encompass a large percentage of women who present for supportive reflexology who are experiencing sub-fertility, and the group is thought to account for up to 25% of women who present for investigation is specialist fertility units. Often the most frustrating diagnosis for women, the rationale presented in this material pertaining to elevated levels of stress hormones relating to the HPA axis might well go some way to better explaining this large group of women.

Repeated miscarriage

It's been estimated that miscarriage occurs in 15-20% of all pregnancies, usually in the first three months. After a woman experiences three or more miscarriages, it's referred to clinically as 'repeated miscarriage'. The causes of miscarriage are varied:

Chromosomal: one of the most common causes of miscarriage, thought to comprise of over 50% of all miscarriages. Potentially, the number of chromosomes in the foetus, the structure of the chromosome, or even the genetic material that they carry may present a problem.

Abnormalities of the uterus such as a double uterus and conditions such as fibroids can sometimes cause problems.

Hormonal imbalances

Immunity problems: sometimes the body can view the foetus as a foreign body and so attacks the pregnancy. Blood tests can sometimes determine if a woman has this immunity problem.

Male sub-fertility

Sub-fertility is thought to affect 1 in 20 men. The results of two sperm samples are normally analysed by the GP, around 6 weeks apart. Male clinical sub-fertility terminology includes:

- Oligozoospermia -Reduced number of sperm
- Asthenozoospermia - Reduced sperm motility
- Teratozoospermia - Increased abnormal morphology in sperm
- Azoospermia - Absence of sperm
- Necrozoospermia - All sperm non-viable or non-motile
- Oligooasthenoteratozoospermia (sperm variable all abnormal) is the most common cause of male sub-fertility. Male sub-fertility is rarely caused by hormonal imbalances, rather lifestyle and environmental factors are thought to impact more directly. In the first instance men are encouraged to make lifestyle changes where appropriate.
- For most couples where male sub-fertility is indicated assisted conception techniques can offer a good chance of conception.

A normal range sperm sample demonstrates:

- 2ml volume - Sperm concentration of >2 million/ml.
- Motility > 50% progressive or 25% rapidly progressive
- Morphology >15% normal forms
- White blood cells <1 million/ml
- Immunobead or mixed anti-globulin reaction test <50% (presence of antibodies coating the sperm)

Clinical interventions in sub-fertility:

Primary (GP) protocols relating to **female** sub-fertility can include:

- Cervical smear
- Test for chlamydia and other STDs
- Ovulation testing: checks progesterone levels seven days before menstruation
- Blood tests to determine hormone levels: including TSH (thyroid stimulating hormone); FSH (follicle stimulating hormone); LH (luteinising hormone) and estradiol levels. FHS and LH tests are generally carried out between day 2 and 6 of the menstrual cycle. These tests can potentially also rule out early menopause.
- Referral to a gynaecological unit or in some cases directly to a specialist IVF unit.

For **men** (GP):

- Sperm test checking morphology (shape), motility (movement) and count.
- Test for Chlamydia

Common secondary protocols for sub-fertility include referral to a consultant gynaecologist or specialist fertility unit for:

A laparoscopic investigation is a commonly used keyhole surgery procedure used to investigate, diagnose (and treat) pelvic abnormalities and clinical conditions such as endometriosis.

Clomifene Citrate is a fertility drug used to stimulate and/or regulate ovulation by blocking oestrogen receptors in the pituitary gland, leading to increased production of FSH. Increased FHS levels in turn stimulate the development of dominant ovarian follicles. Generally clomifene is only prescribed within specialist fertility units because of an additional requirement for uterine ultrasound monitoring; linked to a risk of multiple follicle development and in some cases hyper stimulation of the ovaries.

Intrauterine Insemination (IUI) washes and separates fast moving healthy sperm, returning it to the woman's uterus at the time of ovulation, via the use of a catheter. IUI might be performed stimulated or un-stimulated. When the cycle is stimulated the woman is also given fertility drugs to better ensure ovulation occurs. The success rate of IUI is only slightly higher than that of natural conception.

In Vitro Fertilisation (IVF): IVF involves gathering oocytes (obtained surgically) from ovarian follicles and prepared sperm which are then fertilised outside the body (in vitro means in glass). Embryos derived from these oocytes are then re-implanted in the woman's uterus.

Information is provided here relating to a generic IVF protocol. In reality however, each specialist fertility unit has its own individual way of carrying out the protocol. Some units might start on a particular day of the woman's menstrual cycle; some don't. Some units might administer antibiotics to the women and her partner prior to commencing the protocol; again some don't. Some units might use a nasal spray to down regulate the women in the first phase whilst some might use a pen-injection. Some doctors will 'tweak' the IVF drugs to suit the individual woman; whilst some units may have a one protocol fits all policy. Increasingly units are providing short-protocol IVF: over in less than three weeks. Given the nature of the specialism the IVF protocol is not carried out in every local hospital, and so many reflexology practitioners may only be within range of one or two specialist IVF units. It is essential practitioners gather research regarding their local unit/s individual clinic protocols.

In Vitro Fertilisation (IVF) for women involves:

Step 1: the down-regulation phase

Women administer drugs daily/twice daily (usually GnRH) to suppress pituitary function. Treatment is administered via a nasal spray or a daily injection. Down regulation is principally used in super ovulation regimens to prevent the surge of luteinising hormone and the release of oocytes prematurely.

Step 2: stimulating egg supply

Once the menstrual cycle is successfully suppressed, FSH (follicle stimulating hormone) is administered by injection for approximately 12 days.

Step 3: monitoring

Vaginal ultrasound scans are performed regularly (particularly in the final week of the drug protocol) in order to ensure the woman is responding to the drugs correctly. When the follicles measure a sufficient size (> 18mm in diameter) women are given the go ahead to administer an injection of human chorionic gonadotrophin which helps eggs to mature and occurs around 34-38 hours prior to egg collection.

Step 4: egg collection

Eggs are usually collected by ultrasound guidance, with the woman under sedation.

Step 5: insemination, fertilisation and embryo transfer

Eggs and sperm are mixed and cultured by the embryologist for approximately 16–20 hours. Fertilised embryos are allowed to develop for a further 24-48 hours, before the best embryo(s) are chosen for transfer back to the woman's uterus (normally one or two embryos are returned: numbers are restricted by guidelines because of the risks associated with multiple births). Embryos have usually developed by this stage into four, six or eight cells respectively. In some cases embryos are allowed to develop to blasocyst stage (day 5). Women are required to administer progesterone medication (normally pessaries) for up to two weeks to ensure the lining of the uterus remains in place.

IVF for men: sperm collection

A fresh sample of sperm is retrieved generally at the time of egg collection (unless frozen sperm is being used) and the healthiest sperm then selected for the IVF/ICSI process.

Intra-Cytoplasmic Sperm Injection (ICSI)

An ICSI protocol for a woman is exactly the same as the IVF protocol. The difference lies in the manner in which the egg is inseminated and fertilised. ICSI is a specialist variant of IVF where the embryologist injects a single sperm directly into the cytoplasm of the egg. ICSI is generally carried out when there is a problem with the sperm. This might be connected to poor count, morphology or motility, or it might be as a result of sperm collected post vasectomy, or because sperm has been previously frozen or gathered surgically from the epididymis or testes.

Freezing embryos

Additional embryos cultivated by IVF, measured to be of sufficient quality may be suitable for freezing depending on the individual facilities available to each IVF unit and their associated protocols. Shortened IVF protocols are common place in instances where there are frozen viable embryo's available. Interesting research has demonstrated that the success rates for frozen embryo transfers in IVF patients may be higher than success rates with convention IVF protocols.

Short protocol IVF (Soft IVF)

Short protocol IVF cycles are sometimes utilised in women who are older and perhaps display a lower egg stock, or women who may have not responded well a previous IVF protocol.

More information regarding ART can be found by visiting The Human Fertilisation and Embryology Authority at www.hfea.gov.uk

Common hormone medications

Progestogens

Progestogens are synthetic hormones that behave like the natural hormone progesterone. They stop eggs from being released by the ovaries (ovulation). The mirena coil intrauterine system is a T-shaped contraceptive device that fits into the womb and releases progestogen into the body.

Antiprogestogens

Also known as testosterone derivatives, antiprogestogens are synthetic hormones that bring on an artificial menopause by decreasing the production of oestrogen and progesterone. Side effects can include weight gain, acne, mood changes and the development of masculine features.

Gonadotrophin-releasing hormone (GnRH) analogues

Like antiprogestogens, GnRH analogues are synthetic hormones that can encourage an artificial menopause. They are taken as a nasal spray, implant or injection and work in a similar way to gonadotrophin-releasing hormone (a natural female hormone). Taken continuously for more than two weeks the production of oestrogen is stopped. They often have side effects such as hot flushes, vaginal dryness and low libido, so can often be recommended alongside hormone replacement therapy (HRT), which is usually used to reduce the symptoms of menopause. GnRH analogues are used in the treatment of many sub-fertility conditions, in addition to being used in the IVF protocol.

CHAPTER SIX

RELATIONAL REFLEXOLOGY SUPPORTING SUB-FERTILITY CLIENTS IN PRACTICE

Integration of knowledge - developing the therapists toolbox

Aside from attending relevant continuing developmental courses practitioners can also improve their knowledge base and practitioner 'toolbox' through sourcing relevant specialist reading material, engaging with professional associations, and making use of up to date research papers and past lectures. Practitioners can source useful information relating to holistic and clinical research papers in books and online. It is also equally often very helpful to encourage clients to do their own personal research into topics such as nutrition and diet and even meditation techniques as this promotes and encourages pro-active client participation.

Practitioner use of self

As we explored in chapter four practitioner *use of self* is required in forming effective therapeutic relationships. Within a relational reflexology context and relating specifically to work involving emotional vulnerable and anxious client groups, practitioner use of self might be defined as utilising during sessions any additional appropriate professional skills. Many complementary therapists for example are qualified and well versed in meditation techniques and guided visualization techniques. To complement the reflexology package practitioners are encouraged to utilise such techniques, aiming to promote more instances of focused relaxation. Whilst it is undoubtedly essential adequate professional training accompanies any such additional intervention and that the purpose of any such intervention is solely focused towards the client's needs, the use of such interventions should be utilised and can often prove to be invaluable additional *take home* sources of support.

How much does a relational reflexologist need to know?

Practitioners wishing to engage with sub-fertility clients are ethically bound to demonstrate a high standard in their practice. The duty upon professional reflexology practitioners today is enormous, and the body of informed knowledge required to practice ethically encompasses not only clinical and medical information, but also relational information, modality specific information and is absolutely requiring of a personal holistic overview capable of appreciating the multi-dimensional impact of many health conditions.

Developing a professional personal rationale for practice requires a foundation of sound theoretical understanding underpinning practice in addition to a proficiency in practical the application of the modality. Denise Tiran (2011) believes it is essential professional reflexology practitioners are furnished with a high level of clinical information and should:

> *"understand the pathology related to conditions, and (how) to apply this knowledge to the individual so that treatment can be effective and safe."*

Integrating appropriate levels of informed knowledge is vital for professional practitioners who wish to work with either diagnosed clinical conditions and/or emotionally vulnerable client groups.

Whist it would be entirely unprofessional to engage in any type of clinical work without first acquiring an appropriate level of informed knowledge it would also be fair to state reflexologists are certainly not medical professionals. A consultant endocrinologist undoubtedly will be equipped with a detailed, microscopic knowledge of their specific field of expertise. A GP in practice is equipped with a much broader range of information, spanning all body systems. The GP may possess a working knowledge of the endocrine system, but he is not required professionally to hold the same level of detailed information as the consultant.

Holistic practitioners are required, much like the GP, to be similarly equipped with a broad range of appropriate knowledge, but should think in terms of mind, body and spirit, striving to develop an more in-depth understanding of each relevant component and any potential interactions.

Practitioners should strive to practice in a professional and complementary manner; that being defined as *alongside* the medical profession, with a basic appreciation of medical and clinical terminology therefore clearly essential.

Collectively, professional relational reflexology practitioners should aim to demonstrate:

- A high standard of theoretical comprehension regarding reflexology (form). The ability to professionally apply that theoretical information in practice
- A good understanding of A&P and how it's related to conception and pregnancy
- A good understanding of A&P and how it's related to clinically diagnosed sub-fertility conditions
- A deep appreciation of the emotional strains involved in sub-fertility
- A good understanding of how to build safe and supportive therapeutic relationships

- A good understanding of how stress and anxiety can potentially affect the physiological processes in the body via the HPA axis
- An appreciation of relevant and appropriate nutritional information
- An appreciation of relevant and appropriate client self help techniques

How can reflexology support the sub-fertility client?

- Reflexology and touch promote focused states of relaxation and encourage physiological states of calm in the autonomic system, calming fight or flight responses and dampening the effects of the HPA axis
- A collaborative therapeutic relationship can be formed
- Clients feel understood, safe and supported
- Education, goal setting and the introduction of client focused time promote relaxation and a deeper sense of inner control. Dietary and other wider lifestyle changes promote autonomy and a less stressed, better fuelled, physiological body

The focus of relational practice

The collective and collaborative aim of relational reflexology practice is to promote high states of relaxation in the client. This might sound quite simple really, and within the confines of a forty minute or hour long session of reflexology it is ultimately within reach of nearly every practitioner. The real skill in relational reflexology however lies in the practitioner's depth of knowledge, coupled with precisely how that knowledge is related to, and utilised within, the supportive confines of the therapeutic relationship. Increased instances of the relaxation state are desirable both within and outside of the confines of the weekly sessions. The sessions, the practitioner and the knowledge can be utilised as a weekly metaphorical *spring-board,* used to re-enforce change and positively encourage clients. The deep sense of relaxation induced as a result of attending for professional supportive reflexology can promote feelings of being more grounded thus allowing clients to re-focus positively towards the coming week.

Externalising and building trust - the crucial first session

There are many ways of understanding the concept of *externalising* and one of the most common is *'the person is not the problem, the problem is the problem'*. When a problem becomes *internalised* often an individual can come to believe something is really wrong with them, or believe that *they* are the real source of the problem. Within a counselling context specifically the aim of externalising emotions is therefore to help people realise that *they* and *the problem* are not in fact the same thing.

Within a relational reflexology context externalising naturally occurs simply as a result of increased education. Both educational information and any emotional support gained from the relationship and verbal exchanges can encourage externalisation of problems because the information provides clients with a context in which to make positive changes.

For example, it is not unusual for a woman to report feeling markedly different regarding her sub-fertility situation after the workings of the HPA axis, and the potential effects of fight or flight hormones on human reproduction have been explained properly. Suddenly with this new information a more developed and informed viewpoint can begin to form. This new outlook places the problem into a new and different external context. The client can now start to view herself and her *problem* as more separate entities. As the client starts to make appropriate changes within this new more informed framework, so her feelings and emotions can also begin to alter.

It would be entirely wrong to imagine the vulnerable nature of this client group means the women only use the confines of a reflexology session to cry uncontrollably or reside in a place of sadness and self-pity. On the contrary, whilst these women can indeed often break down and cry during reflexology sessions it is often either near the beginning of a session or towards the end. Crying at the start of the session might be a result of women bottling up their emotions throughout the preceding week, and an emotional pressure cooker effect developing as clients enters what they recognise as a safe space. Crying occurring towards the end of a session can be often result from the physiologically relaxing effects of the reflexology, combined with verbal exchanges and quiet reflective moments, encouraging bottled up emotions to come to the surface.

Universally and overwhelmingly however women experiencing sub-fertility want more than anything to feel pro-actively involved in their journey, and are therefore naturally drawn towards any intervention providing an additional element of personal understanding or control. After all, it is what prompted them to pick up the phone and enquire about supportive reflexology in the first place. Sub-fertility clients generally want to help themselves.

Interestingly a comment often voiced regarding sub-fertility counseling experienced in IVF clinics focuses on a dislike of the sometimes assumed *grief* theme assumed by infertility counsellors. Sub-fertility clients are generally not quite ready to give up and *grieve* when they struggling to conceive or are about to undertake an IVF treatment. Women want to feel positive and feel they are doing all they can to pro-actively ensure success. If and when the time arrives for a client to halt her personal quest and accept natural motherhood is not going to happen for her, she will come to that conclusion independently, and only when the time is absolutely right for her.

For most women however, either natural or assisted conception does occur eventually with an estimated 4% of couples remaining involuntarily childless (Braude & Taylor, 2004). The role of the relational sub-fertility reflexologist is primarily to support women in the here and now, to touch, to care, to educate when necessary and to listen and offer support in those moments required.

Engaging with sub-fertility clients

Women presenting with undiagnosed sub-fertility challenges should be signposted to their own GP in the first instance to rule out any underlying medical conditions which might prevent conception.

For natural sub-fertility client's supportive relational reflexology can be delivered across 12 weekly sessions, or across at least two full menstrual cycles. A session plan should be discussed and agreed upon during the consultation period, and client progress regularly reflected upon with any appropriate alterations made where necessary. The integrative package is designed towards promoting deep states of relaxation. Dietary changes are geared towards the promotion of more balanced blood sugar levels, and therefore a more balanced general endocrine system. Using the supportive nature of the relational encounter clients should be educated regarding their physiological body; therefore giving context for why any changes might be beneficial. The practitioner should strive to offer a safe, warm and supportive space. The choice of how the client uses that space and is hers alone, and the therapist's role is entirely supportive and empathic in essence.

Collectively the work is focused towards promoting a reduction of stress, fear and anxiety, and therefore any associated effects stemming from elevated fight or flight hormones in the body. The sessions aim to promote more instances of base line *relaxation state* therefore the rationale assumes there exists a connection between increased stimulation of the HPA axis and some instances of unexplained sub-fertility.

Engaging with IVF clients

For supportive reflexology in ART specifically, reflexology should commence preferably at least six weeks prior to the start date of the IVF/ICSI protocol. A session plan should be discussed and agreed upon during the consultation period, and client progress regularly reflected upon with any appropriate alterations made where necessary. Initially the focus leans towards supporting the body through the initial down-regulating phase of the IVF protocol: the stage where a woman's body is placed into a state of menopause using powerful hormones. Practitioners should be particularly concerned during this initial phase with promoting stimulation of the blood and circulation. Using the supportive nature of the relational encounter, clients should be appropriately educated regarding their bodies physiological function; therefore giving context for why any changes might be beneficial. The practitioner should strive to offer a safe, warm and supportive space. The choice of how the client uses that space and is hers alone, and the therapist's role is supportive and empathic in essence.

Collectively the work is focused towards promoting a reduction of stress, fear and anxiety, and any associated effects stemming from elevated fight or flight hormones in the body. The sessions aim to promote more instances of base line *relaxation state*; therefore the rationale assumes there exists a connection between increased stimulation of the HPA axis and IVF/ICSI success rates.

Promoting wider self-care - dietary considerations

There are many ways in which the sub-fertility client might choose to focus upon self care. Engaging in any pro-active activity which helps a client to feel more in control and more relaxed can have obvious benefits. Clients often find making more time and restructuring their lives accordingly across the session period to make room for more focused time on self care develop these feelings of being more pro-active and in control. Dietary changes are rarely without benefit to the sub-fertility client. It is often positive to ask clients to personally research any recommended changes, as this stance promotes autonomy and self directed change. Collaborative education however in the first instance might focus upon:

Diet and the endocrine system

The clinical association made for example between the insulin resistance and sub-fertility conditions such as PCOS, serves as a good reminder that both the pancreas and thyroid glands are organs which produce hormones belonging to a much larger and more complex generic endocrine system. The pituitary gland deep in the brain stimulates the thyroid to secrete the hormones responsible for regulating the rate at which the body burns off nutrients to produce energy, and the pancreas is responsible for producing insulin, a hormone enabling the body to metabolise and store carbohydrates. The adrenal gland produces adrenaline when states of anxiety and the fight or flight responses are introduced. When this state occurs the body automatically begins to burn off energy at a vastly increased rate, using that energy to support increased heart rate and blood supply to the muscles.

Consuming regular, nutritionally balanced meals helps to ensure more balanced blood sugar levels are maintained in the body and therefore promotes a more balanced functioning endocrine system in general. Clients who make these changes normally experience increased and sustained energy levels as well as better functioning digestive systems. In the PCOS client specifically, following a type II diabetic diet can facilitate huge changes in the menstrual cycle. Advice and education should be encouraged not only to help with sub-fertility issues but also to ensure improved health across a long term basis.

Poor nutrition

Sufficient levels of magnesium, selenium, zinc, folic acid and vitamins B6 and vitamin E are all considered essential for conception. A healthy balanced diet incorporating regular intakes of fresh fruit and vegetables, pulses, grains, seed in addition to unprocessed carbohydrates and proteins can help better insure good health. Poor nutrition in women experiencing sub-fertility issues often displays in a regular or shortened cycle coupled with a very light or short menstrual bleed. Women in this category often on closer inspection of their diets rarely consume an adequate daily quota of protein.

Protein is utilised by the body to build new cells, maintain tissue and construct new proteins to further support renewal and maintenance of the body systems. Some of the enzymes created by the body as a result of the consumption of protein, such as nucleoproteins (ameno acids and nucleic acids) are essential in the creation of every new cell in the body, as well as the creation of every new human. The body requires over 20 different amino acids to construct all the new proteins required to function normally. Ten are essential amino acids which must be obtained from food. The others are referred to nonessential amino acids and can be manufactured by the body from existing fats and carbohydrates.

Animal proteins are viewed as high quality proteins because they contain a similar combination of amino acids to that of humans. Proteins derived from grain, fruits, vegetable, pulses and nuts and seeds (with the exception being the soya bean) can often contain limited amounts of one or more required essential amino acids.

Making changes in this area specifically will often display quickly as an improvement in bleed quality and duration in the first instance, often followed by a lengthening of the menstrual cycle where necessitated.

Liver function

Reducing toxin build up in the bloodstream through ensuring good quality nutrition should also be viewed as an important consideration regarding general health and sub-fertility. According to TCM the energy associated with the liver is closely associated with the quality and frequency of woman's menstrual bleed. Anatomically, the liver can be likened to the bodies very own chemical processing plant. When we consider much of what the body ingests eventually ends up in the blood stream; and the function of the liver to clean and process the blood, it is easy to understand why considering the *quality* of the foodstuff we consume in the first instance might be important to our health. Foodstuffs heavy in chemical additives and preservatives should be particularly avoided by the sub-fertility client and especially in those women who might be categorised as having dysmenorrhea or menorrhagia.

This is also a particularly important consideration regarding women undergoing IVF. The strain placed on the function of the liver when dealing with powerful IVF drugs in regards to the body's natural instinctive drive towards the elimination of foreign toxins, means it is vitally important that client's try not to place any additional pressure on the organ. Clients who present with particularly unhealthy eating habits, or those who find difficulty in formulating change, should be signposted to a qualified dietician who can provide more detailed advice regarding appropriate nutritional changes.

Calming the stormy mind

In addition to promoting pro-active changes in client's eating habits it can also be helpful to encourage more focused regular instances of relaxation throughout the week. Integrated and utilised regularly, these activities can help to focus the client's mind more in the here and now. Clients who have experienced long term emotional disappointment can often develop a deep inner world, in which they retreat to dwell on their difficult situation.

Frustration stemming from feelings of powerlessness, sadness and hopelessness can lead anxiety and negative automatic thinking patterns developing. It is these feelings which potentially activate the HPA axis and release associated fight or flight hormones.

Understanding the function of the HPA axis and the potential effects of fight of flight hormones can provide clients with meaningful context for change and the concept highlights perfectly the rationale for high levels of practitioner knowledge relating to subjects such as anatomy and physiology and clinically related information.

Sessions should be focused towards encouraging clients back into the here and now and towards better recognising their own physiological *felt sense*. Often through better re-connecting with their physical felt sense clients can begin to feel more in control of their emotional state and can choose to experience their present life in a more conscious manner. For many clients this new perspective is in stark contrast to the dark and lonely world of dealing silently and internally with their sub-fertility issues. The inclusion of interventions such as self hypnosis and guided visualization, and even gentle exercise can all promote these more relaxed states. Additionally the increasingly popular concept of *mindfulness* is an intervention containing many elements helpful for sub-fertility clients.

Understanding mindfulness

Mindfulness as a concept might be described as paying attention in a particular way, on purpose and in the present moment. Developing mindfulness practices can sometimes help clients to overcome and combat negative automatic pilot thinking, which often leads to states of physiological stress and anxiety. The roots of mindfulness lie in Buddhism, but today it has been adapted and is being used increasingly within NHS and business settings, as an intervention to promote wellbeing. Mindfulness practices can include meditation, awareness of breath and body, listening to music or even walking. Mindfulness can be a positive tool for stress management because its principles are easily learned, can be used at virtually any time and can quickly yield positive results. Focused upon learning to calm and quiet the busy human mind, there are many paths which promote mindfulness.

Meditation: Meditation can bring many benefits and has been one of the most popular and traditional ways to achieve a state of mindfulness for centuries. Meditation often becomes easier with practice, but it need not be difficult for beginners. Simply encourage your client to find a comfortable place free of distractions, and begin to quiet her mind. Guided meditations can also be useful for beginners.

Deep breathing: Mindfulness can be as simple as breathing. One of the easiest ways to experience a state of mindfulness is to focus on the breath itself. Breathing from the belly rather than the chest, and trying to breathe in through the nose and out through the mouth. Focusing on the sound and rhythm of the breath, especially when upset can have a calming effect and help clients stay grounded in the present moment. It is impossible to think too much when the focus of the mind is on the breath!

Music: Clients might benefit from listening to soothing slow-tempo new-age or classical music. Focusing on the sound and vibration of the notes and perhaps any feelings the music brings to the surface can help keep clients connected in the experience. If other thoughts creep into the head, clients might simply acknowledge them, gently bringing the attention back to the current moment and the music

Observing thoughts: Many anxious people find it difficult to stop the rapid stream of thoughts running through the mind, and the idea of trying to sit and meditate and hold off the onslaught of thoughts can actually cause more stress. If this sounds like your client, the mindfulness exercise of observing thoughts might be more suited to them. Rather than working against the narrative running in the head, clients can sit back and *observe* the thoughts. As clients begin to observe their thoughts they may find their mind naturally quieting and the thoughts becoming less prominent.

Journaling: Some clients might find journaling a helpful way of processing their thoughts. Often just acknowledging the way we feel by writing it down can help to reduce the intensity of the associated though and any related anxiety.

CHAPTER SEVEN

REFLECTIVE CASE STUDIES

All case study material presented is taken from the writer's real practice. Permission has been sought from each of the women represented and anonymity and confidentiality assured. The studies are presented in qualitative manner so as to better attempt to present and represent the multi-dimensional experiences of each client.

Case Study I: the IVF client

Karen, an otherwise healthy 44 year old professional woman presented for treatment asking to be supported through her upcoming IVF protocol. Karen had already undergone seven full protocol IVF attempts (in addition to one frozen cycle and one IUI cycle) across a number of years. Now divorced, single, and feeling as though her time and opportunities to be a parent were perhaps running out, Karen decided to opt for both donor eggs and sperm. She was to be supported though the initial stages of IVF by a respected UK unit, and her embryo transfer would take place abroad. It might be a fair to say Karen was understandably nervous and worried about the impending IVF. Her previous failures left her emotional drained and familiar with disappointment. Karen was anxious to do all she possibly could to ensure a successful outcome at what would probably be her final attempt at IVF. Karen attended for reflexology for 14 weeks prior to embryo transfer. Across this time she seemed to take particular encouragement from the rationale presented regarding the potential effects of the HPA axis on conception, and this information prompted Karen to start to make more time in her life centred upon better self care, relaxation and promoting calm. Sessions were utilised to draw encouragement and re-assurance from the therapist and Karen seemed to adopt a more philosophical attitude as the weeks went moved on. We'll now turn to Karen's words to try and understand more about what was experiencing:

"I am a 44 year old GP who had been trying to conceive for 8 years. I am pleased that I rang a few months before treatment was due to begin and essentially we had our first consultation on the telephone. (The therapist) spent about 40 minutes asking questions, talking through my history and about her positive experiences of helping women to conceive. At the time of my first appointment (the therapist) spent a further hour and a half with me talking and the performing the reflexology treatment. I felt very relaxed after the treatment, but it was different from other reflexology experiences, where I had fallen asleep for most of it. I felt more alert and found that (the therapist) spent time finding out more about me, my experiences and giving me very positive messages and challenging some of my negative thoughts. I went for reflexology regularly from then on, usually about once a week, but sometimes less frequently. I was advised to increase my protein intake and that would help with energy levels. Over the weeks I was starting to look less tired and wrung out. (The therapist) talked about the negative effect of stress hormones on the uterus and the reduction in the chances of embryos implanting, which made a lot of sense. Because of my treatments I realised how stressed and deflated I had become as a result of the repeated failures. (The therapist) gave me faith that the treatment could work if we got my body and mind in a confident state and ready to receive a pregnancy. I was going to be away in Cyprus for the treatment and (the therapist) was very reassuring that not having reflexology for a couple of weeks would not impact negatively on the outcome, because we had already helped my body and mind into the right place to conceive. With a previous practitioner I would have rushed back up from embryo transfer to have acupuncture, which seemed to add to the stress and the pressure of the whole process. I felt relaxed as I left for the transfer and managed to deal with the whole experience well. I had had so many negative tests previously that fear was stopping me taking the pregnancy test when the time came. I was too scared of the outcome. I arrived for reflexology and (the therapist) without quite saying it told me I was being ridiculous (something my friends had not quite managed to do) and that the outcome would

be the same whether I checked or not, and it may well be positive. I did the test there and then and then sat having reflexology feeling stunned by the positive result and constantly checking the stick that I could not put down. (The therapist) offered that I did not have the treatment as she was sure I had plenty of people to phone but I wanted to have it). A long journey! I am now 32 weeks pregnant with twins - a boy and a girl! Both are to doing well on the scans and are over 3 and a half pounds each. I am sure reflexology has played a significant part in preparing me for this pregnancy and ensuring that my body and mind were in the right place to receive a pregnancy. (The therapists) treatment, support, advice, stories of her life experiences and good humour have all played a vital role in helping me to finally become pregnant. Something that I thought would never happen. I am eternally grateful."

Clearly from a quantitative standpoint there are several different factors in this case which might have individually and/or collectively contributed to Karen's positive result; not limited to the use of donor eggs and sperm; the embryo transfer taking place abroad; the inclusion of supportive reflexology and even increased levels self care. It would be impossible to quantify the effect of each factor however it might be fair to state existentially, the benefits of supportive reflexology for Karen seem clear and demonstrable from her words.

Case study II: the IVF client

Joanne, an otherwise healthy 34 year old woman presented for reflexology after the failure of her second IVF attempt. Joanne's Mother, so concerned about her daughter's wellbeing sourced supportive reflexology and encouraged her daughter to attend for hoping the sessions might help induce relaxation. Emotionally and physically it would be fair to say Joanne was utterly exhausted. It was decided collaboratively between practitioner and client that initially the sessions would be focused towards attempting restore Joanne's general health and well being; rather than focusing on pregnancy or another IVF attempt. Joanne's words:

"After two failed IVF cycles I felt very emotional, I felt it was all my fault and although my husband and I were in it together I felt so alone, and no longer felt like a woman, but more

like a machine going through a process. My family became very concerned about me as they could see I was struggling and they knew I needed help to cope. My parents looked on the Internet as they'd heard reflexology might be excellent for my needs.

My therapist just understood me: I'd become a shadow of the person I used to be. Because of the sessions I'm much more relaxed and now feel ready to begin another cycle of IVF. I believe supportive reflexology has helped me cope with the day to day stresses and worries that life brings, as well as preparing me for another IVF."

Case study III: the IVF client

Cassie, an otherwise healthy 31 year professional woman, presented for treatment wishing to be supported through an upcoming third ICSI cycle. Cassie had been trying to conceive for five years and prior to starting IVF had been treated pharmaceutically with both clomifene and metformin, in addition to undergoing an ovarian drilling procedure; three unstimulated and two stimulated IUI procedures. Cassie presented weekly for treatment for two months prior to the start of her third ICSI cycle. In Cassie's words:

"I'd always been sceptical of complementary therapies, all the yin and yang, funny smells and gobbledegook terms, but this was something different. Never before had I met a person before who instilled such positivity. For the first time in a long time I felt like someone finally understood me, understood our situation and genuinely wanted to help. Her down-to-earth and truthful approach was something we hadn't experienced during treatment so far. Everything else was very generic, and we were just a number in a very large group with a common theme; unexplained infertility. The therapists approach was different; she dug deep to learn more about me as a person and alongside the reflexology the work was heavily complemented by a genuine desire to learn about the feelings I was experiencing, and the desire to try to unravel the negative thoughts spinning round in my head. After my first session, I genuinely had a lot of respect for her work: not only did she clearly know her subject areas, but she also respected the views I held, and the concerns that had developed over my medical treatment. Throughout the coming weeks I learnt to open up about things I'd never really shared before, and own up to the feelings I had; laying them on the table and mentally smashing the negative ones with a huge hammer. Rather than concentrating on the thoughts placed in our minds by our medical professionals, I began to realise that all the

inconclusive testing was actually a positive thing. My mindset changed and it was no longer about consultants not being able to find a real cause for our constant failures, it became more about the fact that they couldn't find a cause because there just wasn't anything wrong; there was no reason for the treatments not to work. This became my new outlook. The NHS waiting times between treatments were long but I used this time to let (the therapist) work her magic and get me into the most positive and relaxed mindset possible. Don't get me wrong, there were still moments I sat quietly on a night and asked myself if I was living in the real world, or was I letting myself be led into a place where fairies danced and where everything was going to be nice and perfect. Physically, my menstrual cycles started to change and became less of a hassle. My partner was finally able to take his tin-hat off and felt safe I wasn't going to throw things at his head every month. As our final IVF cycle loomed, I actually felt more in control than I had throughout any other treatment. My partner and I made all the decisions around our treatment; not the nurses, nor the consultants. I was in a positive place and didn't experience the pressure I'd felt on myself during other cycles. January 2013 was a new start and our treatment went relatively smoothly, just as the previous cycles had. The outcome though was unexpected. After over 60 months of unbearable disappointment, seeing a single blue line each and every time, we finally saw 2 very definite blue lines. Now, at 18 weeks, with 2 strong beating hearts and a beautiful rounded bump we feel utterly blessed. The pain and heartache of the last few years is still fresh in our minds, but the feeling of joy as the flutters begin makes everything so worth it. We are incredibly lucky, and don't take anything for granted at the moment but this amazing feeling of waking up each morning knowing our lives are changing in such a wonderful way is a feeling that cannot be put into words. As for the yin and the yang, the funny smells and the gobbledegook; which actually makes perfect sense, we're now firm believers. To be understood as person, rather than counted as an unwanted statistic makes every difference".

Case study IV: the unexplained sub-fertility client

Esther, an otherwise healthy 36 year old woman, presented for treatment hoping to be supported in her desire to become pregnant for the third time after recently having experienced miscarriage. Esther was anxious to add to her family, particularly wanting to conceive a sibling for her young son, and it would be fair to say for feelings of panic had set in. Over the coming weeks Esther made changes to her diet (ensuring to eat regularly to promote balanced bloods sugar levels and ensure restorative energy supply) whilst the reflexology sessions were focused towards drawing encouragement and support from the therapist. In Esther's words:

"After nearly three years of trying to conceive my cycle was a bit of a mess and my emotions were all over the place. I had managed to conceive a few times, but each had led to an early loss. My head was in a knot of thoughts that would go round and round, so loud and noisy it was hard to sleep or think straight and everything seemed to come back to one thought; will I have another baby? I started reflexology desperate for some relief from the symptoms of clomifene and hopefully to increase the chances of getting pregnant. I think more than anything I hoped that the reflexology might just help me feel a little more peaceful. I had reflexology once a week and we talked through my feelings, and how I was dealing with things. I found the hour long sessions provided intense relaxation, and it would lead to a better night's sleep. At home I followed the advice to improve my diet, but the best thing I was advised to do was to be kind to myself. I focused on what would make me feel better and what I enjoyed. After the first month of treatment the flow of my period was much improved, and didn't feel so congested. The PMT symptoms were reduced and instead of taking multiple high strength pain killers, I only needed two tablets across my whole period; which hadn't happened since I was 13. I attended for reflexology for four months and during that time my moods continued to improve, my husband, a non believer in alternative therapies even commented that I was 'better to do with'. I felt a freedom in my mind that allowed me to see things more clearly. I began to believe in my body; that it could and would get pregnant. I even spent my saved up IVF money on a new car! I got a new job to help reduce stress, but before I could even start the new job two lines appeared on a pregnancy test! Reflexology helped me stay calm and relax during the anxious first few weeks, and at eight weeks pregnant I had my first scan and saw two little hearts beating away. Now at 28 weeks both are growing well and weigh 2lb 9 each, we are really looking forward to their arrival."

Case Study V: The unexplained sub-fertility client

Sophie, an otherwise healthy 36 year old woman, presented for treatment hoping to be supported in her desire to conceive. Sophie reported a history of long and irregular menstrual cycles since stopping the birth control pill a number of years before. Already having unsuccessfully undertaken six sessions of stimulated IUI treatments, Sophie felt IVF was her only chance of conception. In the three months running up to the start of the IVF process, reflexology was administered weekly and changes were introduced to the diet to promote increased protein consumption and more balance blood sugar levels (Sophie was a naturally slender, tall lady who carried little excess weight). Sophie's previously extended cycle was reduced to 28 days and she started to menstruate regularly and consistently, demonstrated by changes to bleed quality and duration. In Sophie's words:

"Two weeks prior to my IVF start date, I discovered I had conceived naturally. I firmly believe I would never have achieved this without (reflexology). I found the treatments to be extremely beneficial and left after each appointment feeling refreshed and relaxed."

Case study VI: the IVF client (blocked fallopian tubes)

Elaine, a 38 year old woman presented after having suffered with dysmenorreah for many years, latterly coupled with anovulation. Further tests had confirmed the presence of blocked fallopian tubes and Elaine had already had 3 unsuccessful attempts at IVF. Focus of treatment was primarily towards promoting relaxation and better self care in an attempt to reduce feelings of fear and anxiety regarding Elaine's upcoming and final attempt to conceive a child through IVF. Elaine's words:

"At the first treatment I explained my circumstances. (The therapist) knew what was required. I felt she understood me!! I received 9 weeks of Reflexology before the IVF cycle and continued throughout. I am convinced the treatments helped me to conceive. I was mentally and physically prepared. Reflexology helped me to be more positive and I felt less stressed. I know we would not have achieved our dream without it".

Elaine has subsequently gone on to conceive a second child with the help of IVF and was supported throughout by reflexology.

Case study VII: The endometriosis client

Jane a 35 year old woman presented after a friend recommended reflexology. Jane was suffering from severe endometriosis: after three largely unsuccessful laparoscopies was still experiencing extreme pain and exhaustion and struggling to return to work after a year off sick. Jane had been informed by her consultant that natural conception was unlikely, although the thought of embarking on IVF treatment was still far in the future for Jane. Her immediate concern was pain. A plan was constructed which included making dietary changes in an attempt to promote less strain on liver function (blood and menstrual problems link directly to liver function, according to the principles of TCM) as well as introducing more protein and fluids. At the first session the pathology of Jane's feet was acutely sensitive, and the pressure therapy deeply uncomfortable in some areas, despite very gentle finger and thumb movements. Over the weeks this acute sensitivity lessened, directly in line with an improvement in Jane's general pain levels and an associated reduction in the use of topical analgesia (thus promoting a less stressed liver). Jane's words:

"After an intensive course of reflexology I found I was better able to deal with my pain levels and felt emotionally stronger. I returned to work four days a week, fairly quickly. Within three months of starting the treatments I was delighted to find I was pregnant. I would recommend reflexology to anyone experiencing similar problems. I am convinced I would never have felt better, nor fallen pregnant without (it)."

As is fairly common in some women with endometriosis, pregnancy and a period of breast feeding resulted in a vast reduction of Jane's returning symptoms post pregnancy. Jane continues to uphold her dietary considerations and promote good circulation in an attempt to reduce the symptoms returning.

Case study VIII: hormonal imbalance (preventative sub-fertility)

Gillian, a 27 year old woman presented for treatment asking for support connected to a suspected hormonal imbalance. Since stopping the contraceptive pill two years prior, Gillian had suffered from a multitude of distressing symptoms, including dry hair, an irregular menstrual cycle and worsening cystic acne and emotionally she reported feeling low lethargic, anxious, depressed and unfeminine; Gillian was also concerned about her future fertility. Blood tests had been performed by her GP who suspected PCOS however post ultrasound scan, it was decided that Gillian did not meet the appropriate diagnostic criteria for PCOS. Feeling there was no feasible course of action left within conventional medicine, Gillian presented for supportive reflexology:

"I haven't looked back since my first appointment. (The therapist) suggested some straightforward lifestyle changes and I felt more positive even after the first week. I felt supported by someone who understood me. Three months later I felt completely back to normal. My menstrual cycles returned to a more regular pattern, my skin is well-behaved and clear, my hair stronger and shinier and I had more loads more energy ! Not only did (the therapist) educate me using her knowledge base in complementary therapies, she has proved a warm, empathic and inspiring force who has given me my quality of life back. My sessions were always uplifting and encouraging and with (the therapists) guidance, I have now set a precedent for how I will always now listen to and respect my body"

The supportive environment of a practitioner's therapy room can also be educational when supported by sound knowledge. PCOS (Gillian is displaying many of the identifying symptoms associated with PCOS) is linked to insulin resistance in the body. Making simple alterations, such as following a type II diabetic diet can result in huge changes across many physiological and emotional areas for the PCOS client.

Having the dynamics of an endocrine system explained can suddenly bring enlightenment to the client who may have been wondering why a simple thing like dietary changes might affect the much wider systems of the body. Most clients when quizzed have no idea what the function of the liver is for example, or how the food we consume might affects it's function, nor do clients often understand the pancreas secretes a 'hormone' called insulin and that hormone belongs to the very same endocrine system that regulates their ability to conceive. Education brings empowerment to the client and empowerment can encourage positive change.

Case study IX: the repeated miscarriage client

Paula, an otherwise healthy 31 year old woman presented for treatment after experiencing two miscarriages over a two years period. Paula heard about reflexology from a friend and thought it might help. Despite an obvious improvement in Paula's fertility rate across the treatment period (she became pregnant and miscarried a further three times across a 12 month period), Paula and her husband crushed by yet another disappointment, eventually concluded emotionally and physically their journey to conceive naturally had come to an end. Paula and her husband have subsequently gone on to adopt two beautiful children and as a family today they could not be happier. In Paula's words:

"It is hard to sum up in a few words how much treatment helped me when I was going through my journey to becoming a parent, but here goes! Physically I felt after each consultation that I was completely relaxed (driving home was always a bit of an effort!). Throughout the duration of the treatment I did become pregnant several times but sadly these pregnancies were not meant to be. Emotionally, when I first met (the therapist) it was like speaking to an old friend but someone who really understood what we were going through and truly empathised. I had confidence (in the treatment) but never assumed that the outcome would be a baby, even though that's was what we hoped for. In the end we have two beautiful boys, through adoption. I believe that in attending for reflexology treatment regularly (the therapist) kept my mind in good health, which kept me in a position to adopt. Trying to have a family is all consuming and it can be hard to see anything outside that when you are stuck in the middle of it – (reflexology) managed to achieve that. I will always be eternally grateful for all the help and support on our journey even though we are not good for baby statistics!!! I am so pleased our journey has been what it is. I have never been so happy and proud to be a mum of our two gorgeous, loving sons – this was our path and (reflexology) helped us on our way."

Despite her painful difficulties Paula's experience remains entirely valid example of why supportive reflexology can benefit sub-fertility clients. Paula experienced increased levels of fertility across the session duration, despite the further sad loss of these pregnancies (possibly owning to genetic factors given a similar gestation period at which each of the pregnancies was lost) demonstrates reflexology can help women conceive naturally. Paula's experience though also perhaps importantly demonstrates the huge supportive and emotional benefits gained from engaging with a confident and empathic reflexology practitioner. Therapeutic support stemming from the application of reflexology is perhaps well demonstrated in this case as extending far beyond the pressure therapy alone.

Undoubtedly the practitioner's role in this case study involved heavy ethical responsibility. The practitioner although confident to re-engage post an appropriate recovery period, only did so after appropriate and careful discussion with the client. It was the client who led the way, owning her own experience and the practitioner's role was entirely supportive.

Case study X - Ruby - the unexplained infertility client

Ruby an otherwise healthy 34 year old woman presented for treatment after suffering several months of constant heavy menstrual bleeding. Ruby was waiting to start ICSI due to a problem with her husband's sperm complicating her sub-fertility issues. In the three months running up to the ICSI start date Ruby attended for reflexology weekly. Ruby conceived naturally a few weeks prior to her ICSI start date. In Ruby's words:

"Instead of obsessing about possible reasons for not conceiving, reflexology focused on the physical and mental issues that had put my body in turmoil and supportive reflexology gave me a sense of perspective and hope. Stopping the contraceptive pill after 14 years left me with constant bleeding and hormonal irregularity, so that my body felt completely alien to me. Reflexology helped me to reclaim and understand my body, so that within weeks of starting treatment, I was healthier and happier than I had been in years. It took less than 10 weeks to prepare me to conceive naturally. Throughout the pregnancy, reflexology kept me grounded, focused and healthy. One of the most valuable aspects of (the therapists) approach is her understanding that it is not possible to completely remove all potential barriers to conception. Giving up a stressful job was not an option for me, but the treatment helped me to understand how my body responded to that stress, and therefore gave me the power to choose a different response. I maintain that reflexology 'got me pregnant', and

have recommended (it) to friends in similar situations. I wish that every woman battling fertility issues could be lucky enough to benefit from such therapy; to ensure a successful outcome, and to equip them with a true knowledge of their bodies during pregnancy, birth and the ensuing hormonal maelstrom."

Case study XI - Jacqui - the unexplained sub-fertility client

Jacqui an otherwise healthy 29 year old woman presented wishing to be supported with ongoing sub-fertility issues. Jacqui already had a seven year old daughter and had been trying to conceive for over two years. As is common for women experiencing sub-fertility issues who have already conceived a child Jacqui considered reflexology as a viable option before embarking along the very expensive private IVF route. (Free NHS fertility treatment (ART) is not generically available to women who have previously conceived a child or where a partner has previously conceived a child). Jacqui expressed her deep frustration and emotional distress clearly during her first session and explained how she longed to give her daughter a sibling and experience pregnancy herself once more. In Jacqui's words;

"I initially decided to try reflexology following a friend's recommendation. I was due to have surgery to remove a damaged fallopian tube and wanted to try and be in the best place possible to conceive afterwards. I had been trying for my second child for two and a half years and had been informed by Doctor's IVF would be the only way to conceive. My husband and I were reluctant to go through this expensive process, knowing there was no guarantee of success. Straight away at my initial consultation (the therapist) put my mind at ease with her positive, confident approach. After my op and recovery period, I started to attend weekly sessions. I went in very open minded believing I had nothing to lose and everything potentially to gain. The therapist's approach - straight up and combined with humour, meant I found I looked forward to the sessions and loved the reflexology; it was so relaxing. I tried to look at things more positively: telling myself I would be pregnant very soon. Before long I honestly felt the best I had in a long time. Be the end of the intensive period of weekly sessions I was due my period but had also been feeling different with weird symptoms. Not knowing what to think I took a pregnancy test and found I was pregnant! I couldn't believe it and after only eight sessions of reflexology! I now go once a month for reflexology as I feel it is so beneficial to my wellbeing. I would seriously tell anyone to open

their mind to complementary "alternative" therapies such as reflexology as I feel people such as me are perfect examples to show they definitely help. Don't remain a doctor's statistic; broaden your mind".

Clearly in Jacqui's case the removal of her malfunctioning fallopian tube will undoubtedly have factored considerably in potentially increasing the possibility of natural conception occurring. However, Jacqui's words also demonstrate the wider existential benefits she felt were gained from attending for sessions.

Summary and reflection

When reflecting on the words of the women the existential value derived from receiving supportive relational reflexology seems to have been experienced as wholly beneficial to the health and well-being of this particular client group. *Support, advice* and *education* seem to be some of the most highlighted benefits identified, as well as feelings and sense of being *understood*. *Better sleep* and *relaxation* are also mentioned often, as well as feeling more *positive*.

The experiences presented in these case studies gives context for the relational reflexology rationale for professional practice which states; aside from the benefits of a touch pressure therapy, supportive reflexology has much to offer to the general public and in particular emotionally vulnerable client groups, such as the sub-fertility group. Practiced to a high professional standard, holistically, ethically and mindful of the delicate interacting processes connecting mind and body, supportive relational reflexology has proven to be immensely beneficial to each of these women.

The women's words also perfectly highlight the deep frustrations often experienced, and how emotional vulnerability is common place amongst many sub-fertility clients. High levels of practitioner competence and sufficient levels of self development are therefore of paramount importance.

This is probably this most important; most all encompassing event, ever to take place in a woman's life. As practitioners of relational reflexology we must respect that all important fact and ensure at all times our clients remain safe, and are cared for with the utmost respect.

Sub-fertility is not a field of holistic dreams, nor is it one filled with magic or false promises. Supportive relational reflexology is a professional and ethically driven field requiring only excellence, honestly and genuineness. Human interactions, touch, support and knowledge are the collective elements responsible for any 'magic' taking place. Women make the changes that *really* matter and the professional practitioner's role is to demonstrate, through the medium of reflexology, touch and the supportive therapeutic relationship how those changes might be made.

CHAPTER EIGHT

OBSERVATIONS AND STATISTICS IN PRACTICE

Physiological changes noted to the menstrual cycle in sub-fertility clients

Clinical evidence gathered from within the writer's private practice supports a time frame of approximately three full menstrual cycles for change to occur physiologically: relating to twelve weekly reflexology sessions – the depth, speed and effectiveness of the changes noted are unsurprisingly linked to the level of change made directly by the client. Statistically only women diagnosed with PCOS take longer to demonstrate change in the menstrual bleed (up to 16 weeks depending on the severity of the disorder and the presence of insulin stabilisers).

The menstrual bleed is one of the few physiological indicators a reflexologist can utilise to ascertain change in the hormonal cycle. Therapists should become interested in examining verbally the bleed during the consultation; making note of frequency, duration, colour, and flow across the days. Menstrual pain and discomfort should also be noted, as well as any other classical symptoms associated with PMS, such as lethargy, breast tenderness, emotional outbursts, acne, headaches and migraines or changes in regular bowel movements. These 'symptoms' should be tracked weekly throughout changes and noted during the catch up consultation each week. Positive reflection on the changes occurring in the presenting symptoms of a client can be a powerful stimulating force to encourage clients to keep looking forward with an open mind.

Reflexology supporting the women through IVF

Clinical observations within the writer's private practice have demonstrated that that application of reflexology (combined with dietary changes) during the down-regulation phase of IVF can reduce side effects most commonly noted during the protocol. These include headache and migraine, hot flushes and night sweats and emotional outbursts.

Clients who present for reflexology for the first time who are undertaking their second or third attempt at IVF can often report a reduction in the frequency and severity of the side effects, often also line with increased egg numbers at the time of retrieval.

Working through ovulation, conception and beyond

Clinical observations gathered from within the writers practice have demonstrated that the application of reflexology across both ovulation and conception will do no harm. To date the writer has worked with over 150 women (combined natural sub-fertility and supportive ART Clients). The writer's success rate (to live birth) stands at over 80%. In each and every case work has continued with these women using reflexology until such a time as the clients feel safe and ready to disengage from treatment (normally around the 8-12 week scan point for IVF clients, and 6-8 weeks for natural sub-fertility).

It is not the writer's opinion that the application of reflexology will in any way effect negatively the development of a well structured, healthy pregnancy.

Noted pathology of the feet in sub-fertility clients

PCOS: The feet and ankles have the tendency to be swollen, cold to the touch and pale in appearance, with deep areas of hardened skin on the plantar region of the foot and dry patches extending up the lower legs. The feet can be difficult to work, with little 'give' present in the tissue.

Endometriosis: Often the over-riding factor demonstrated in the pathology of feet of these women is extreme sensitivity, particularly in the associated pelvic and reproductive areas. Long before women have enquired as to what that area relates to its common to find clients wincing in pain at what your thought was your most gentle of finger movements. Over time and with regular treatments this sensitivity seems to lessen, directly in line normally with an improvement in the bleed quality and a lessening of pain generically. The ovary, uterus, bladder and adrenal reflexology points demonstrate the most sensitivity.

Unexplained Infertility: In some women, particularly those women who might be underweight, following a particularly poor diet or anxious, the feet can demonstrate a weakness of tone and poor temperature. Colour seems to be rarely affected. Often as the weeks go by and the diet is improved, *life* seems to come back to these feet again, directly in line normally with an extension of the menstrual bleed duration where required. The feet become warmer and firmer to the touch.

General pathology of the feet

It is very common to find large deep granular deposits at the ear reflexology point. This area also corresponds to an energetic linking point between the TCM kidney and bladder meridians on the foot.

It is common to find deep, granular deposits in the reflexology lung area points. The lung links emotionally to anxiety, over-thinking and stress according to TCM and women with deposits in this area when questioned will often confirm waking during the night; describing their mind as racing and busy.

It is not uncommon to find swollen and protruding big toe pads (head and brain reflexology points). This is perhaps reflective of the over-thinking associated with stress. Additionally in this area it is often common for clients to feel a definite 'sharp' sensation when the pituitary reflex point is worked and for the therapist to be aware of a more pronounced point, physiologically.

In women experiencing dysmenorrhea it is not uncommon for the feet to sweat excessively throughout treatment for approximately 4-5 weekly sessions. This phenomenon often also occurs in women suffering with conditions such as fibromyalgia, chronic migraine and adult acne. This may potentially be linked to sluggish liver function, with the stimulation resulting from the reflexology triggering the body's autonomic use of the skin as a secondary supportive detoxification organ.

Swelling occurs across the pelvic lymph area of the foot and ankle approximately four days prior to menstruation. Approximately two days prior to menstruation a band of heat (notably warmer than the temperature of the rest of the foot and leg) forms across the pelvic lymph area. The affected area extends from the ovary point, across the top of the foot and ankle and ending near the uterus point on the inside of the foot. This band of head will last until at least the end of the first full day of bleeding, but generally not past the second day.

Pathology of change in the feet relating to the menstrual cycle

It is possible to estimate where a relatively normal hormonally functioning woman is in her menstrual cycle by examining the pathology of the feet.

When the ankle appears slightly swollen and both ovary points feel as though the tip of your most sensitive finger is able to rest comfortably in a natural curve, the client is likely to be in the third week of her menstrual cycle.

When the ankle is hot and swollen the woman is about to start menstruating or has just begun to do so.

When the ankle appears normal in temperature and displays no fluid retention and both ovaries points feel as though the tip of your most sensitive finger rests comfortably in a natural curve, then woman is likely to be finishing her bleed and moving into the second week of her menstrual cycle.

When the ankle appears normal in temperature and shows no fluid retention and one or both ovary points feel hardened to the fingertip then ovulation is likely to be occurring.

Table 1.1: Statistic in Practice Relating to Sub-Fertility and Supportive ART

Natural Sub-Fertility	Client Total	Live Births	%
(Unexplained Sub-Fertility)	19	15	78.9%
PCOS	3	2	66.6%
Endometriosis	5	3	60%
(Supportive ART)	Client Total	Live Births	%
IUI	3	1	33.3%
IVF	106	86	81.1%
ICSI	12	8	66.6%

Note: women are often unsure whether fertilisation took place via IVF or ICSI

Natural Supportive Sub-Fertility:

20 women from a total of 27 became pregnant during or shortly after an intensive course of supportive relational reflexology (12 weeks minimum) demonstrating a success rate of 74% generically.

Of the 20 women all 20 were receiving supportive reflexology for the first time.

Supportive ART:

95 women from a total of 121 became pregnant undergoing ART whilst receiving supportive reflexology, demonstrating a 78.5% success rate generically.

Of these 95 clients 86 are receiving supportive reflexology for the first time and 9 are undertaking a second supportive relational reflexology cycle.

Of the 95 women who went to live birth (IVF/ICSI): 45 are on 1st cycle ART, 37 are on 2nd cycle ART, 8 are on 3rd cycle ART, 4 are on 4th cycle ART and 1 is one 8th cycle ART.

Of the 95 women who went to live birth (IVF/ICSI) one received donor egg and sperm.

Of the 95 women who went to live birth (IVF/ICSI), 81 women had single pregnancies, 1 woman gave birth to triplets and 13 women gave birth to twins.

CHAPTER NINE

A BRIEF INTRODUCTION TO TCM (TRADITIONAL CHINESE MEDICINE)

Eastern attitudes relating to health and the nature of the universe have remained relatively unaltered across many thousands of years. An absence of any influence stemming from classical Greek thinking means Eastern ideas and concepts have remained much closer to their ancient, mystical origins. Initially dismissed on mass by Western thinkers as simply philosophical and ethnological traditions, it was sadly assumption alone which suggested Eastern traditions were fundamentally scientifically flawed and defective.

Eastern philosophies however are universally clear in stating that both time and space are inseparably connected, with each other and other aspects of the universe, such as the concepts of movement and energy. Interestingly, Eastern philosophies are presently being viewed by many modern physicists as corresponding and aligning much more closely to modern scientific thinking than was ever imagined possible.

Traditional Chinese medicine dates back to around 2900 BC and was said to be founded by the part mythical creature Fu Hsi, who first described the concept of Qi and the universal principles of yin and yang. Indications stemming from writings such as the Huang Ti Nei Ching (The Yellow Emperor's Treatise on Internal Medicine c. 770-467BC) demonstrates clearly

early Chinese cultures believed man to be a perfect image of the cosmos and absolutely attuned to nature,

"Man instinctively and collectively understood and lived in accordance with its fundamental forces" (Graham, 1990).

At the heart of TCM lies the tenet stating the root cause of illness, not just the symptoms must be treated. TCM offers a truly holistic approach acknowledging every aspect of a person, their body, mind, and spirit as part of one complete interacting dynamic, as opposed to loosely connected pieces to be treated individually.

A TCM interactive perspective on health:

- Disease, illness, weakness and emotional extremes
- Deficiency, excess or stagnation of energy (QI) in a TCM organ system
- Imbalances in the associated physiological organ system of the body
- Susceptibility to experiencing emotional responses

Reflexology and TCM

The first writings referencing and foot diagnosis in Chinese culture can be found in the Huang Ti Nei Ching. As TCM gradually developed a more complete and detailed medical system, hand and foot diagnosis unfortunately failed to develop alongside more commonly known diagnostic tools; and therefore foot massage remained a relatively minor branch of TCM until the time of the Ming and Qing Dynasties, when the physician Hau Tuo (145-208AD) coined the form *'Zu Xin Theory'*.

"Because of the simplicity and practicality (hand and foot massage) has long been very wide spread among the ordinary people of China, although it was not admitted to the honoured

ranks of classical tradition of medicine due to certain historical reasons." (Genwei & DongFang, 2006)

During the Ming and Qing Dynasties TCM massage was developed and combined with the theory of meridians and acupoints. Points on the hands and feet were frequently used within TCM massage in the treatment of diseases. In the book 'Hao Tuo Cheats' it states:

"massaging the foot in spring strengthens immunity; in summer relieves heat; in autumn prevents constipation and in winter warms the body.

Today in China reflexology is practiced within the holistic principles of TCM, and is combined with the clinical experience of modern medicine.

According to the ancient Chinese there are meridians or energy pathways which run all through the body and each meridian is linked to various organs and functions. When the Qi in the body is able to run through the meridians smoothly and unhindered, good health prevails. When it becomes blocked or obstructed illness occurs. Therefore treatment according to TCM is principally concerned with normalising energy flow in the body.

There are 23 acupoints on the hand; 9 on the palm and 14 on the top of the hand associated with the lung, large intestine, heart and small intestine meridians.

The foot acupressure points are believed to reflect various disease states in the body. It is believed disease states can be alleviated by massage because of an intimate relationship between the feet, the viscera *(internal organs)*, the meridians *(energy pathways)* and the blood.

There are 33 acupoints located on the foot associated with the stomach, spleen, bladder, kidney, liver and gallbladder meridians. Within TCM the feet are viewed as a fundamental source for treatment and regarded as the *roots* of the human body.

The three treasures in TCM - life sustaining energies

Jing - nutritive essence, essence; refined, perfected; extract; spirit, demon; sperm, seed

The Chinese word for 'essence', specifically referring to the kidney essence; the Jing is said to be the material basis for the physical body. The Jing nourishes, fuels, and cools the body and is the carrier of our genetic heritage. The production of semen in males, and menstrual blood (and pregnancy) in females are believed to place huge strains on the levels of Jing in the body.

Given individuals are said to be genetically gifted with a finite amount of Jing, the efficient replenishing of energy in the body is of paramount importance according to TCM in maintaining good health. According to TCM the restorative energy required for maintaining good health is sourced from food Qi (see figure 1.2) and prolonged by breath Qi (exercise and meditation). The Chinese therefore believe healthy Jing is not only important regarding conception, but also in maintaining longevity in the individual.

Qi - vitality, energy, force; air, vapor; breath; spirit, vigor

Qi can be translated as vital energy that when free flowing and unrestricted, reflects in a healthy body. Qi flows through pathways called meridians and is most associated with the liver and and spleen systems. Qi animates our bodies, allowing movement; the movement of breath in and out of our lungs and the movement of blood through the vessels. In TCM blood is considered as a fluid not only confined to blood vessels, but also runs through the meridians of the body.

Shen - spirit; soul, mind; god, deity; supernatural being

Shen or 'spirit' resides in the heart and mind. A healthy, vibrant person is described as having good Shen and it is often considered to be reflected in shining and twinkling eyes; viewed as an emanation of spiritual radiance and an enlightened and forgiving heart and mind.

Metaphorically if we try to imagine Jing as the wax and wick of a candle and Qi its flame, then Shen might be seen as the radiance given off by the flame. In the same manner as the light from the candle is dependent on wax, wick and flame, so healthy *Shen* is dependent on the cultivation of good Jing and Qi. A balanced and healthy body and mind therefore enables the radiant spirit to shine.

Understanding Qi

According to TCM Qi is the fundamental energy of nature and the universe. Each movement or change in the physical world can be related to movement and changes of Qi. Similarly, everything that happens inside the body is driven by the flow of Qi. TCM theory states in order to maintain good health the body must have enough Qi and the Qi must be free to flow throughout the body smoothly, thus ensuring all the vital organs and tissues are supplied with the energy required to function correctly.

If levels of Qi in the body drop due to poor nutrition or because of heightened emotional states, or if the flow of Qi becomes blocked or hindered, the body can become susceptible to experiencing *dis-ease* and poor health within the body systems.

Jing (source Qi): The Jing is inherited genetically at conception. Source qi resides in the kidney and from there flows throughout the body via the meridian system. Source Qi provides the vital organs with the energy to function properly and efficiently. Source Qi requires nourishment which is obtained from essential Qi.

Essential Qi: This nourishing Qi forms when Qi from the lungs and Qi from food essence combine. The essential or pectoral Qi is stored in the chest and has two principle purposes; to support the heart (circulation) and lungs (respiration).

Defensive Qi: This Qi is formed from food essence and provides immune support for the body. It resides in the muscles, skin and hair. Defensive Qi holds the ability to regulate the skin for example, helping to control the temperature of body tissue.

Nutrient Qi: This Qi again originates from food essence. Nutrient Qi resides and circulates in the blood vessels, and is responsible for generating new blood and for nourishing existing blood as it is circulated by the body.

Zang Fu theory

According to the tradition of TCM the theory of zang-fu defines the composition of internal organs as well as the energy systems that link each organ to one another, and in turn to the whole of the body. The theory describes the production, transformation, and maintenance of the four basic life materials (essence, Qi, blood and body fluids) by the zang fu organs. The study of any zang-fu organ system includes both the physiology of the specific organs as well as their related tissues. States of dis-ease might be explained as conditions of excessive, deficient, or stagnant energy (Qi) within the zang-fu organ system.

The yang organs function to transform and store Qi are associated with the interior of the body. The fu organs function to clear the body of waste and associated with the exterior of the body. Table 1.2 outlines the main and associated organs belonging to each paring with its related sensory organ and emotion and the wider related systems and functions. Closer inspection of the organ associations listed in figure 1.2 demonstrates the correlation between a balanced and nutritious diet and the energy required by the body to hold and nurture new life. The energy of the liver and kidneys for example (with associated links to the blood/uterus (liver) and conception (kidney) are replenished by spleen energy which is linked directly to the food we consume.

Seven emotions in TCM

One fundamental difference existing between TCM and a Western allopathic view of health might be the inclusion of and importance placed on emotions in the individual are how emotions are intertwined within the principles of good health and medicine. The Zang-Fu associations also demonstrate that certain organs are related to emotional responses, for example, the heart is related to joy; the liver to anger; the spleen to pensiveness; the lungs to anxiety and the kidneys to fear. According to TCM therefore excessive emotional states can be considered as a major internal cause of dis-ease.

Emotional activity is generally considered as a normal physiological response to stimuli from the external environment. Within ordinary conditions and presented with more ordinary stimuli, emotions are not considered to induce illness or weakness in the body.

However, when emotions become elevated and prolonged in their duration the individual can become prone to injury occurring in internal organs and therefore more susceptible to dis-ease. Whilst Western medicine tends to stress the more psychological aspects of psychosomatic ailments, the pathological consequences of emotional states on the internal organs is conversely of primary concern to the TCM practitioner. The seven emotions according to TCM are:

Joy: In TCM, joy refers to a state of agitation or overexcitement, rather than passive happiness. Over-stimulation of joy can lead to problems associated with the heart and is connected with feelings of agitation, insomnia and palpitations.

Anger: Anger according to TCM encapsulates a whole range of emotions including resentment, irritability, and frustration and it's believed an excess of rich blood can encourage anger in the individual. Anger is believed to affect the liver primarily resulting in a stagnation of liver Qi, leading to liver energy rising to the head often resulting in headaches, and dizziness and even high blood pressure and can cause problems. The liver meridian is also believed to run directly through the uterine cavity and is believed to be responsible for providing a woman's menstrual bleed each month.

Anxiety: Anxiety is believed to cause injury to the lungs according to TCM and shallow and irregular breathing are considered a symptom of anxiety. The shortage of breath experienced during periods of anxiety is common to everyone. Anxiety also causes problems in the fu organ associated with the lung: the large intestine. For example, over-anxious people are prone to ulcerative colitis and IBS.

Pensiveness: According to TCM, pensiveness is considered to result from thinking too much or excessive mental stimulation and the organ most at risk is the spleen. A deficiency of spleen Qi can also result in feelings of worry fatigue, lethargy, and an inability to concentrate.

Grief: Grief, according to TCM is also associated with the lungs. Unresolved chronic grief can create disharmony which in turn is believed to interfere with the lung's function of circulating Qi around the body.

Fear: Again fear is considered as a perfectly normal human emotion, however when fear becomes chronic and the perceived cause cannot be directly addressed, then disharmony is believed to occur in the kidneys. In cases of extreme fright, the kidney's ability to hold Qi may be impaired leading to involuntary urination.

Fright: Fright is distinguished from fear according to TCM by its sudden, unexpected nature. Fright is considered to initially affect the heart but if it persists it can become a more conscious fear and move to the kidney.

Sub-fertility, emotions and TCM

The spleen, liver and kidneys energies are clearly important organs according to TCM whenever considering sub-fertility issues. It is worth noting according to TCM, unless there is a mechanical or anatomical reason which prevents conception taking place, sub-fertility does not exist, instead there is considered to exist an unbalanced system, with conception viewed essentially as a perfectly natural element of being a healthy human being.

Associations between the emotions of fear and fright and kidney energy, in addition to the fluctuating energy of the spleen for example highlights the importance of encouraging and promoting increased states of relaxation and calm in women experiencing sub-fertility issues. Excessive emotions might be considered to *eat up* vitally required energy according to TCM and so the practice of meditation and focused energetic practices such as Qigong are widespread in the East. Activities such as these are utilised primarily to encourage more instances of calm in the mind and to promote the cultivation of vital energy. In fact Qigong translates literally as *life energy cultivation.*

Women experiencing sub-fertility issues can often report experiencing strong emotions of fear, anxiety, panic, frustration and even anger. According to TCM fear and anxiety are associated with kidney energy, and the kidney further associated with reproductive hormones and the ability to conceive. Therefore helping women to reduce feelings of fear, according to TCM, can help to maintain energetic vitality and strength in the vital kidney energy responsible for human conception.

Table 1.2: Zang-Fu Table

Zang Organ	Associated Fu Organ	Sensory Organ	Associated Emotion	Associated Systems and Functions
Spleen	Stomach	Mouth	**Pensiveness**	*Spleen energy is responsible for extracting nutrients from the food we consume and converting those nutrients into blood and Qi. Meridian active between 7-9am & 9-11am. Linked to the stomach and upper part of the digestion. Mouth ulcers, sickness (reversed Spleen/stomach Qi is often associated with excessive emotions and a feeling of having something stuck in the throat impeding any feeling of being hungry.*
Liver	Gall Bladder	Eyes	**Anger and agitation**	*Associated with the blood and **free flow of blood and qi around the body (circulation),** liver function and **toxin removal** (the liver might be likened to a chemical processing factory), Meridians active between 11pm-1am & 1-3am. Associated with muscles (containing blood), the eyes, **menstruation (liver 'gives' blood to the uterus each month).** Links to headaches and migraines. fibromyalgia, Poor circulation and the tendons*
Kidney	Urinary Bladder	Ears, genitals and anus	**Fear and fright**	***Houses the 'Jing' (or life force energy) required for life and conception.** Regulates the kidneys and urinary system. Meridians active between 3-5pm & 5-7pm. **Associated with fright, fear and exhaustion.** Links to the ears and so associated with vertigo, tinnitus and labyrinthitis. Regulates the elimination of toxins, the bones, hair, and **reproductive hormones**.*
Lung	Large Intestine	Nose Skin	**Anxiety and grief**	*Linked to asthma, chest infections, IBS, eczema, rashes and flaky dry skin. Meridians active between 3-5am and 5-7am. The lung energy supports the heart and circulation and can be easily depleted as a result of stress or over-thinking. When lung energy is disturbed because clients are stressed they may have the tendency to wake around 4am (when the meridian is most active).*
Heart	Small Intestine	Tongue	**Joy**	*Linked to the vessels and vascular problems palpitations, chest discomfort, insomnia. sadness, anxiety issues, shyness, vascular Meridian active between 11am-1pm & 1-3pm*

GLOSSARY OF CLINICAL AND RELATIONAL TERMINOLOGY

Amenonorrhea:

The generic term used to refer to the absence of a woman's menstrual period.

Anovulation:

The generic term used to refer to a lack of ovulation in a woman.

ART:

Assisted Reproductive Techniques.

Autonomy:

n. Philosophy - the doctrine that the individual human will is or ought to be governed only by its own principles and laws.

Autonomy is important within a therapeutic context because the concept is central to promoting self-directed change in clients.

Beneficence:

The principle of beneficence means acting in the best interests of the client based on professional assessment. It directs attention to working strictly within one's limits of competence and providing services on the basis of adequate training or experience.

Ensuring that the client's best interests are achieved requires systematic monitoring of practice and outcomes by the best available means. An obligation to act in the best interests of a client may become paramount when working with clients whose capacity for autonomy is diminished because of immaturity, lack of understanding, extreme distress, serious disturbance or other significant personal constraints.

Congruence:

n. Agreement, harmony, conformity, or correspondence.

Within a therapeutic context congruence can be defined as one of 'ways of being' linked to the core conditions proposed by the humanist psychologist and founder of person-centred counselling, Carl Rogers (1951). Congruence refers to state of being in which the practitioner attempts to be present herself as more 'real' and present in the relationship.

Disclosure:

n.. The act or process of revealing or uncovering.

Within a therapeutic context disclosure refers to the personal and emotional material clients choose to bring to the consulting room.

Dysmenorrhea:

The generic term used to describe excessive menstrual pain.

Empathy:

n. Identification with and understanding of another's situation, feelings, and motives. Empathic understanding demonstrate the practitioner's ability to appreciate the client's unique frame of reference

Endometriosis:

A medical condition in which cells from the lining of the uterus (endometrium) appear and often grow outside of the uterine cavity.

Existential:

adj. 1. Of, relating to, or dealing with existence.

2. Based on experience; empirical.

Externalising:

tr.v. 1.To attribute to outside causes.

2. To project or attribute (inner conflicts or feelings) to external circumstances or causes.

Within a therapeutic context *externalising* can help clients to re-define their stance and provide context for self-directed change.

Homeostasis:

n. the tendency of a system, especially the physiological system of higher animals, to maintain internal stability, owing to the coordinated response of its parts to any situation or stimulus tending to disturb its normal condition or function.

2. a state of psychological equilibrium obtained when tension or a drive has been reduced or eliminated.

HPA Axis:

The hypothalamic-pituitary-adrenal axis is a complex set of interactions between the hypothalamus (brain), the pituitary gland (brain) and the adrenal or suprarenal glands (at the top of each kidney.)

The HPA axis helps regulate temperature, digestion, immune system, mood, sexuality and metabolism. It's also a major part of the system that controls reactions to stress, trauma and injury.

IVF:

In Vitro Fertilisation.

ICSI

Intra-Cytoplasmic Sperm Injection.

IUI:

Intrauterine Insemination.

Laparoscopy:

A commonly used keyhole procedure used for investigation, diagnosis and treatment in sub-fertility.

Male Sub-Fertility:

Oligooasthenoteratozoospermia (all sperm variables abnormal) is the most common diagnosis of male-sub-fertility. Sperm tests check sperm count, morphology (shape) and motility (movement).

Menorrhagia:

The generic term used to describe heavy menstrual bleeding.

Multi-Dimensional:

adj. Of, relating to, or having several dimensions.

Within a relational reflexology context multi-dimensional is used to contextualise both the phenomenological experience of sub-fertility client and also the various elements identified within the reflexology package as potentially influencing and therefore promoting change in clients.

Non-maleficence:

Non-maleficence involves: avoiding sexual, financial, emotional or any other form of client exploitation; avoiding incompetence or malpractice; not providing services when unfit to do so due to illness, personal circumstances or intoxication. The practitioner has an ethical responsibility to strive to mitigate any harm caused to a client even when the harm is unavoidable or unintended.

Oligomenorrhoea:

The generic term used to refer to an irregular menstrual cycle in a woman.

PCOS:

Poly Cystic Ovarian Syndrome: a common female endocrine disorder in female of reproductive age.

Person-Centred Theory:

Person-Centred Therapy (PCT) was developed by the humanist psychologist Carl Rogers in the 1940s. The theoretical core of PCT leans towards practitioners developing a more 'personal' relationship with their client. Person-Centred theory promotes the concept than clients are the only experts in their own life.

Phenomenology:

n. A philosophy or method of inquiry based on the premise that reality consists of objects and events as they are perceived or understood in human consciousness and not of anything independent of human consciousness.

Psychoneuroimmunoendocrinology or psychoneuroimmunology:

The study of interactions between psychological factors, the central nervous system, and immune function, as modulated by the neuroendocrine system.

The study focuses on emotional and other psychological states which can affect the immune and endocrine systems, potentially rendering the patient less or more susceptible to disease and triggering autonomic responses.

Relational:

adj.

1. Of, or arising from kinship.

2. Indicating or constituting relation.

Relational Depth:

"A state of profound contact and engagement between two people, in which each person is fully real with the Other, and able to understand and value the Other's experiences at a high level"

Sub-Fertility:

Primary Sub-Fertility: a delay for couples with no previous pregnancies.

Secondary Sub-Fertility:

A delay for a couple who have previously conceived. In some cases the pregnancy may not have been successful (ectopic pregnancy or miscarriage).

Therapeutic Relationship:

A working or helping professional alliance.

Tubal Sub-Fertility:

The generic term used to describe physiological damage to, or loss of, the fallopian tubes.

Unconditional Positive Regard:

A phrase coined by humanist Carl Rogers. UPR can be defined as:

Total acceptance and support of the individual regardless of what the individual says or does.

Unexplained Sub-Fertility:

The generic term used when no clinical cause can be found for sub-fertility difficulties.

CONTACTS AND RESOURCES

Practitioners wishing to expand their skills set in Reflexology may find the following contact information useful:

The Association of Reflexologists (AoR)
www.aor.org.uk

The AoR provide information relating to reflexology training, CPD courses and provide an online member list for the general public

The Clinical Association of Reflexologists (CAR)
www.clinicalreflexology.org

The Clinical Association of Reflexologists provides reflexology training and a member list for the general public

Relational Reflexology Training
www.relationalreflexology.co.uk

Relational Reflexology Training offers advanced CPD reflexology training to experienced practitioners.

Practitioners wishing to source professional supervision may find the following contact information useful:

The British Association of Counselling and Psychotherapy (BACP)

www.bacp.co.uk

The National Register of Psychotherapists (UKCP)

www.psycotherapy.org.uk

More information regarding ART can be found by visiting:

The Human Fertilisation and Embryology Authority
www.hfea.gov.uk

BIBLIOGRAPHY

Balk, J., Catov, J., Horn, B., Gecsi, K., & Wakim, A. (2009). The relationship between perceived stress, acupuncture, and pregnancy rates among IVF patients: A pilot study. *Elsevier*.

Beddoe, A. E., & Lee, K. A. (2008). Mind-body interventions during pregnancy. *Journal of Obstetric, Gynecological and Neonatal Nursing*.

Beddoe, A. E., Paul Yang, C. P., Kennedy, H. P., Weiss, S. J., & Lee, K. A. (2009). The effects of mindfulness-based yoga during pregnancy on maternal psychological and physical distress. *Journal of Obstetric, Gyne and Neonatal Nursing*.

Birk, T. J. (2000). The Effects of massage Therapy Alone and in Combination with Other Complementary Therapies on Immune System Measures and Quality of Life in Human Immunodeficiency Virus. *The Journal of Alternative and Complementary Medicine*.

Braude, P., & Taylor, A. (2004). *ABC of Sub-Fertility.* London : BMJ.

Christian, L. M. (2012). Physiological reactivity to psychological stress in human pregnancy: Current knowledge and future directions. *Elsevier*.

Culhane, ,. J., Rauh, V., Farley-McCollum, K., Hogan, V., Agnew, K., & Wadhwa, P. D. (2001). Maternal stress is associated with bacterial vaginosis in human pregnancy. *Elsevier*, 730.

Daruna, J. H. (2012). *Introduction to Psychoneuroimmunology.* Academic Press.

DeAngelis, T., & Mwakalyelye, N. (1995). The power of touch helps vulnerable babies thrive. *APA Monitor*.

Demyttenaere, K., Nijs, P., Evers-Keibooms, G., & Koninckx, P. (1994). Personality Characteristics, psychoneuroendocrological stress and outcome depending upon the etiology of infertility. *Gynecol Endocrinol*.

DiPietro, J., Mendelson, T., Williams, E. L., & Costigan, K. (2011). Physiological Blunting during pregnancy extends to induced relaxation. *Elsevier*.

Field, T., Hernandez-Reif, M., & Diego, M. (2005). Cortisol Decreases and Serotonin and Dopamine Increase Following Massage Therapy. *University of Miami School of Medicine*.

Fox, S. (2008). *Relating to Clients. The Therapeutic Relationship For Complementary Therapists.* London: JKP.

Galton, G. (2006). *Touch Papers: Dialogues on touch in the psychoanalytic space.* London: Karnac.

Gambles, M., Crooke, M., & Wilkinson, S. (2002). Evaluation of a hospice based reflexology service: a qualiative audit of patient perceptions. *Eur. J. Oncol. Nurs*.

Geib, P. (1998). *Touching in psychoanalytic practice.* Wellington: The New Zealand Psychological Society.

Genwei, W., & DongFang, H. (2006). *Traditional Chinese Hand and Foot Massage.* Beijing: Foreign Languages Press.

Graham, H. (1999). *Complementary Therapies in Context.* London: JKP.

Haugh, S., & Paul, S. (2008). *The Therapeutic Relationship, Perspectives and Themes.* PCCS.

Hazel, C., & Perez, R. (2011). *What Happens When You Touch The Body? The Psychology of Bodywork.* Authorhouse.

Jang, S. H., & Kim, K. H. (2009). Effects of Self-Foot Reflexology on Stress, Fatigue and Blood Circulation in Premenopausal Middle-Aged Women. *Korean Acad Nurs* .

Jourard, S. (1966). An exploratory study of Body-Accessibility. *British Journal of Social and Clinical Psychology* .

Kessler, R. C., Soukup, J., & Davis, R. B. (2001). The use of complementary and alternative therapies to treat anxiety and depression in the United States. American Journal of Psychiatry.

Makereth, P., Booth, K., Hillier, V., & Caress, A. (2009). What do people talk about during reflexology? Analysis of worries and concerns expressed during sessions for patients with multiple sclerosis. *Complementary Therapy Clin.*

Manheimer, E., Zhang, G., & Udoff, L. (2008). *Effects of acupuncture on rates of pregnancy and live birth among women undergoing in vitro fertilisation: systemic review and meta-analysis.*

March-Smith, R. (2005). *Counselling Skills for Complementary Therapists.* London: Open University Press.

Mate, G. (2003). *When The Body Says No. The Hidden Cost of Stress.* Toronto: Vintage Canada.

McLoud, J. (1998). *A Introduction to Counselling.* Buckingham: Open University Press.

Mearns, D., & Cooper, M. (2005). *Working at Relational Depth in Counselling and Psychotherapy.* London: Sage.

Mearns, D., & Thorne, B. (2007). *Person-Centred Counselling in Action, 3rd Edition.* London : Sage.

Mitchell, A., & Cormack, M. (1998). *The Therapeutic Relationship in Complementary Healthcare.* Edinburgh: Churchstone Livingstone.

Paslow, R., Morgan, A. J., Allan, N. B., Jorm, A. F., O'Donnell, C. P., & Purcell, R. (2007). Effectiveness of complementary and self-help treatments for anxiety in children and adolescents. *Medical Journal of Australia* .

Prior, J. C. (1997). Ovulatory Disturbances: They Do Matter. *Canadian Journal of Diagnosis* .

Quattrin, R., Zanini, A., Buchini, S., Turello, D., Annunziata, M. A., Vidotti, C., et al. (2006). Use of Reflexology foot massage to reduce anxiety in hospitalized cancer patients in chemotherapy treatment: methodology and treatment. *Journal of Nursing Managment*.

Rogers, C. (1986). *A Client-centred/Person-centred Approach to Therapy. In Kirschenbaum & Henderson (Eds).* London: Constable.

Rogers, C. (1951). *Client-Centred Therapy.* London: Constable.

Rutter, P. (1989). *Sex in the forbidden zone.* New York: St. Martins Press.

Salvatore, P., Gariboldi, S., Offidani, A., Coppola, F., Amore, M., & Maggini, C. (2001). Psychopathology, personality and marital relationship in patients undergoing in vitro fertilisation procedures. *Fertil Steril*.

Sapolsky, R. M. (2004). *Why Zebras Don't Get Ulcers, 3rd Edition.* New York: St. Martins Press.

Smith, E., Clance, P., & Imes, S. (1998). *Touch in Psychotherapy, Theory, Research and Practice.* New York: Guilford.

Stenzel, C. L., & Rupert, P. A. (2004). Psychologists' use of touch in individual psychotherapy. *Psychotherapy: Theory, Research, Practice, Training*.

Thorne, B. (2002). *The Mystical Power of Person-Centred Therapy.* London: Whurr.

Tiran, D., & Mackereth, P. A. (2011). *Clinical Reflexology. A Guide to Integrative Practice 2nd Edition.* London: Churchstone Livingstone.

Trousdell, P., & Uphoff-Chmielnic, A. (1997). Making Connections. User perceptions of the effects of reflexology and counselling. An evaluation of a complementary health care project at Worthing Mind Report. *Worthing Mind*.

Tune, D. (2001). Is Touch a Valid Therapeutic Intervention? . *Counselling and Psychotherapy Research, BACP*.

Uphoff-Chmiielnik, A. (1999). An exploration into touch in search of a rationale for its use within and as an adjunct to psychotherapy, with an emphasis on a person-centred model; or Beware - Here There Be Tiggers! *Unpublished MA Dissertation, City University London*.

Urich, R. S., Simons, R. F., Losito, B. D., Fiorito, E., Miles, M. A., & Zelson, M. (1991). Stress recovery during exposure to natural and urban environments. *Journal of Environmental Psychology*.

Wadhwa, P. D. (2005). Psychoneuroendocrine processes in human pregnancy influence fetal development and health. *Elsevier*.

Williams, S., Clarke, D., & Gibson, K. (2011). *The Use of Touch in Psychotherapy, A Thematic Analysis.* Germany: Lambert.

INDEX

2546786R00106

Printed in Germany
by Amazon Distribution
GmbH, Leipzig